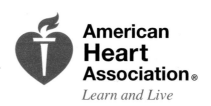

American Heart Association®

Learn and Live

Heartsaver®
Pediatric First Aid CPR AED
STUDENT WORKBOOK

Editors

Louis Gonzales, BS, LP, *Senior Science Editor*

Michael W. Lynch, NREMT-P, *Content Consultant*

Senior Managing Editor

Sue Bork

Special Contributor

Susan Fuchs, MD

First Aid Subcommittee 2012-2013

Jeff Woodin, NREMT-P, *Chair*

Rita Herrington, FNP, *Immediate Past Chair, 2009-2011*

Kostas Alibertis, CCEMT-P

Nate Charlton, MD

Gustavo E. Flores Bauer, MD, EMT-P

Peter Fromm, MPH, RN

John Gonzales, LP

Michael Hendricks, EMT

Helen McCracken, RDH, MS

First Aid Subcommittee 2011-2012

Jeff Woodin, NREMT-P, *Chair*

Rita Herrington, FNP, *Immediate Past Chair, 2009-2011*

Kostas Alibertis, CCEMT-P

Michael A. Buldra, MEd, NREMT-P

Nate Charlton, MD

Jeffrey D. Ferguson, MD, NREMT-P

Gustavo E. Flores Bauer, MD, EMT-P

Peter Fromm, MPH, RN

John Gonzales, LP

Michael Hendricks, EMT

Scott Larson, EMT

Helen McCracken, RDH, MS

David Parish, MD, MPH

Jeanette Previdi, RN-BC, BSN, MPH

© 2013 American Heart Association

ISBN 978-1-61669-260-5

Printed in the United States of America

First American Heart Association Printing July 2013

10 9 8 7 6 5 4 3 2 1

i

> To find out about any updates or corrections to this text, visit **www.heart.org/cpr**, navigate to the page for this course, and click on "Updates."

Contents

CPR, AED, and Choking   93

Preface

Welcome to the American Heart Association Heartsaver® Pediatric First Aid CPR AED Course. This course provides a framework for learning basic skills that may save a life or prevent further injury of an infant or child. The AHA is dedicated to decreasing death and disability when an emergency occurs. The AHA believes that *you* can make a difference. We thank you most sincerely for taking this course.

Our thanks go to the many volunteers and staff who made this course possible. There are not words to express the gratitude felt for their passion, expertise, and countless hours of work.

Jeff A. Woodin, NREMT-P, FAHA
First Aid Subcommittee Chair

Introduction

Welcome to the Heartsaver® Pediatric First Aid CPR AED Course.

In this course, you'll learn both first aid and CPR. In the classroom, you'll watch a video. The video will show you how to give first aid and CPR and help you practice skills. An instructor will coach and test you. If you can give first aid and CPR, you'll be better prepared for an emergency and better able to help save a life.

Using This Workbook

Use this Student Workbook in the following ways:

Before the course:

- Read this Student Workbook.
- Look at the pictures.
- Take notes about policies and procedures. For example, if you work in a child care center that has established policies and procedures for emergencies, review these documents and take notes about how this information will apply to you.

During the course:

- Keep the Student Workbook close by, because it is used at several points during class.

After the course:

- Review the skills frequently.
- Look at the action tables and skills summaries in the Student Workbook (and Quick Reference Guide). This will help you remember first aid, CPR, and automated external defibrillator (AED) use.

How Often Training Is Needed

You need to retake this course every 2 years to get a new course completion card.

Testing and Course Completion Cards

You'll be tested on CPR and on 4 different skills in first aid. Each first aid skill on the test is listed in the workbook as a Skill You Will Demonstrate. You'll find a skill summary sheet listing every skill you'll be tested on at the end of the First Aid section and at the end of the CPR modules. If you demonstrate the skills correctly, you will receive a course completion card.

The information contained in this book is not intended as a substitute for professional medical advice. Please consult your healthcare provider for diagnosis or treatment of any medical conditions.

First Aid

Introduction: First Aid

First Aid Steps

First aid is the help you can provide before someone with more advanced training arrives and takes over. There are 4 steps you need to remember in First Aid. You'll learn how each of these steps works, and then you'll learn how to put it all together in an emergency. The 4 first aid steps are as follows:

Step 1: Prevent	Keeping children from getting hurt is the first step in giving first aid.
Step 2: Be Safe	This is one of the most important ideas in first aid: you have to keep yourself safe if you want to help someone else. You can't help if you're hurt.
Step 3: Phone 911	Knowing how and when to phone for help is one of your best tools. You can give first aid, but sometimes a sick or hurt child needs more help than you can provide. That's when you call people with more advanced training.
Step 4: Act	A child who acts sick usually is. Often, you may know something is wrong but not be sure exactly what that is.
	Looking for and recognizing the problem is one of the most important actions you can take. It helps you figure out exactly what's wrong.
	Once you know what's wrong, you can help.

First Aid Testing

In addition to knowing the 4 steps above, you'll see and practice some specific skills. After practice, you'll be tested. The skills you'll be tested on are

- How to Take Off Gloves
- Finding the Problem
- How to Stop Bleeding and Bandaging
- Using an Epinephrine Pen

These 4 skills are actions you can take to make a big difference.

Step 1: Prevent

Definitions and Key Facts

One of the best ways to prevent injury is to watch children carefully. If you watch them, you may be able to see an accident coming and stop it (a child reaching for a hot pan, for example).

At least half of all fatal injuries can be prevented by simple actions in the home, car, child care center, school, and playground.

Some children with special needs may use special medical devices. A child with diabetes, for example, may have an insulin pump. If you have a child with special needs in your care, learn about what devices the child uses, if any.

What You Will Learn

You'll learn about how to create a safer environment and how to prevent some common injuries.

At the end of the First Aid section, you'll find a checklist you can use to help prevent accidents and injuries.

Topics Covered

- Indoor Prevention
- Outdoor Prevention
- Car Safety and Prevention

Indoor Prevention

What You Will Learn

In this section, you'll learn how to help prevent indoor injuries and reduce the risk of SIDS.

Definitions and Key Facts

It's usually better to phone 911 before Poison Control if a child swallows, touches, or breathes in something that might be poisonous. There are 2 reasons for this:

- A 911 dispatcher can send help right away if needed
- A 911 dispatcher can connect you to Poison Control if needed

SIDS (sudden infant death syndrome) is the sudden death of an infant under 1 year of age that is not explained by other causes.

In the United States, SIDS is the leading cause of death among infants 1 to 12 months of age.

Although the overall rate of SIDS in the US has decreased since 1990, rates for some ethnic groups are still higher than expected.

Action: Indoor Prevention	▪ Post the poison control center number (1-800-222-1222) near a phone where you keep other important information.
	▪ Keep children away from things that can hurt them, including cleaning supplies.
	▪ Install smoke and carbon monoxide detectors and keep working batteries in them.
	▪ Install window guards to keep windows from opening completely.
	▪ Make sure that the building number is visible from the street in case emergency personnel need to find it.
	▪ Make an action plan for emergencies.
	▪ Keep children away from medications and other household items that a child could swallow, such as cleaning supplies and lamp oil.
	▪ Watch children near water. Infants and young children can drown in bathtubs and toilets.
	▪ Never shake or play roughly with a baby. Shaking or tossing a baby in the air while playing can cause serious injury.

For a more complete checklist of things you can do to increase indoor safety, see the Child and Infant Safety Checklist.

Action: Reducing the Risk of SIDS	▪ Put the infant to sleep on her back.
	▪ Make sure the bed only has a mattress, bottom sheet, and the baby.
	▪ Infants can suffocate when they sleep with another person, including a sibling.

To reduce the risk of SIDS, use the Child and Infant Safety Checklist.

Outdoor Prevention

What You Will Learn	In this section, you'll learn how to prevent outdoor injuries. Also see the Child and Infant Safety Checklist.

Definitions and Key Facts	▪ Many childhood injuries happen on the playground and while children are playing organized sports.
	▪ Ideally, parents/guardians will check with a child's healthcare provider before the child starts to play a new organized sport. The child needs to be healthy enough to play.
	▪ Infants and young children can drown in lakes and pools and also in buckets, in only a few inches of water.

Action: Outdoor Safety and Prevention

- Have children wear helmets and safety gear when appropriate.
- Never leave a child alone near water.
- Pools should have fences with 4 sides.
- Have children wear life jackets when appropriate.
- Protect children from too much sun.
- Have children wear closed-toe shoes.
- Clean up any broken glass or trash that could hurt children.

Car Safety and Prevention

What You Will Learn

In this section, you'll learn about car safety and prevention. For more information, see the Child and Infant Safety Checklist.

Definitions and Key Facts

Car crashes are a leading cause of death among children aged 4 to 11 years.

A car seat should

- Fit the child
- Fit the vehicle
- Be installed correctly
- Be used correctly
- Be used every time the child is in the vehicle

Action: Car Safety and Prevention

- Everyone should wear seat belts.
- Everyone should keep arms and legs inside the car.
- Never leave a child alone in the car.
- Select a car seat based on your child's age, height, and weight.
- Install car seats correctly.
- Keep your child in the car seat for as long as possible, as long as your child fits the seat's height and weight requirements.
- All children under 13 should ride in the back seat.
- Children should cross streets at crosswalks and learn street crossing safety.
- Children should hold hands with or be carried by an adult in a parking lot or anyplace cars are moving and drivers might not see a child walking.

FYI: Installing a Child Safety Seat

A child safety seat is safe only if you have installed it properly. Learn how to properly install the safety seat. In your community, you may find child passenger safety experts in some or all of the following places:

- Fire station
- Police department
- Local emergency medical service
- Highway patrol
- Hospital
- Insurance company

Step 2: Be Safe

Definitions and Key Facts

You can't help anyone if you are sick or injured yourself. Keep yourself safe and keep the hurt or sick child safe too.

Hand washing is the most important thing you can do to protect yourself. Another way to protect yourself is to wear gloves.

Taking gloves off correctly is also important, and many people do it incorrectly.

You need to know how to take gloves off without getting blood or body fluids on yourself, so that you can stay safe.

In every situation, you should make sure the scene is safe. Wear gloves, eye protection, and masks whenever appropriate.

What You Will Learn

You'll learn how to keep yourself and the sick or hurt child safe.

Topics Covered

- Assessing the Scene
- Washing Hands
- Universal Precautions
- Exposure to Blood
- Taking Off Gloves (*Skill You Will Demonstrate)
- First Aid Action Plans and First Aid Kits

Assessing the Scene

Definitions and Key Facts

You may have to give first aid in dangerous places. The child may be in a room with poisonous fumes, on a busy street, or in a parking lot.

Before doing anything else, make sure the scene is safe for you and the child. Keep looking around to make sure that the scene stays safe. You can't help anyone if you're injured yourself.

Action: Assess the Scene

As you approach the scene, consider the following:

Danger: Look out for danger to you and danger to the injured child. Move the child only if she's in danger or if you need to move her to provide first aid or CPR. Move her if you can do so safely.

Help: Look for people who can help you, and look for telephones. Have someone phone 911. Phone for help yourself if no one else is around.

Who: Who's injured? Figure out how many people are hurt, and see if you can tell what happened.

Where: Where are you? Be specific. The 911 dispatcher will want to know your address, floor, or location in the building or on the property.

FYI: Know Your Limits

When you give first aid, know your limits. Don't become another victim.

Washing Hands

Definitions and Key Facts

Hand washing is the most important step in preventing illness. Always use soap and water after taking off gloves.

Wash your hands after you give first aid so that you don't spread germs.

Action: Washing Hands Well

Step	Action
1	Wet your hands with clean running water (warm if available) and apply soap.
2	Rub hands together and rub all surfaces of hands and fingers for at least 20 seconds.
3	Rinse hands with lots of running water.
4	Dry your hands with a paper towel or air dryer. If possible, use your paper towel to turn off the faucet.

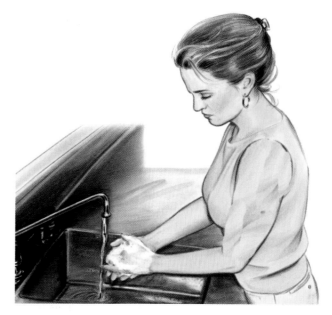

Figure 1. Wash your hands well with soap and water after giving first aid.

Important

Use a hand sanitizer if you can't wash your hands with soap and water. Rub your hands well to loosen germs, and then allow the sanitizer to air dry.

Universal Precautions

Definitions and Key Facts

Universal precautions are called "universal" because you should treat all blood and blood-containing materials as if they contain germs that can cause diseases. These safety measures are precautions intended to protect you and everyone else.

Protect yourself from touching blood or something that has blood on or in it. That's the best way to keep from becoming sick because of the germs in blood that can cause disease.

For those who are required to use personal protective equipment (PPE), such as teachers and child care workers, you need the following equipment:

- Gloves to protect your hands from blood and other body fluids that contain blood
- Eye protection, if the child is bleeding, to protect your eyes from blood and other body fluids
- Mask to protect you when you give breaths

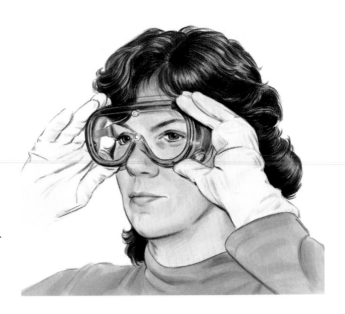

Figure 2. Wear PPE provided by your employer when it is appropriate or required by your employer.

Action: Protecting Yourself From Blood

Treat all blood and anything that has blood on it as if it does have germs that can cause diseases.

Step	Action
1	Wear PPE whenever required or appropriate.
2	Place all disposable equipment that has touched blood or body fluids containing blood in a sealed waste bag (or do what your child care center requires).
3	Follow your center's plan for disposing of waste that has blood or anything with blood on it.
4	Wash your hands well with soap and lots of water after properly taking off your gloves.

Exposure to Blood

Definitions and Key Facts

Bloodborne diseases are caused by germs. A rescuer may catch a disease if germs in someone else's blood or body fluids enter the rescuer's body, often through the rescuer's mouth or eye or a cut on the skin. To be safe, rescuers should wear PPE—gloves and eye protection— to keep from touching the injured child's blood or body fluids.

Three examples of bloodborne diseases are

- Human immunodeficiency virus (HIV), the virus that causes AIDS
- Hepatitis B
- Hepatitis C

Action: Exposure to Blood

Step	Action
1	If you are wearing gloves, take them off.
2	Immediately wash your hands and the contact area with soap and lots of water.
3	If body fluids have splattered in your eyes, nose, or the inside of your mouth, rinse these areas with lots of water.
4	Tell your supervisor what happened as soon as possible. Then contact a healthcare provider.

Taking Off Gloves (*Skill You Will Demonstrate)

Definitions and Key Facts

- When you give first aid, the outside of your gloves may touch blood or other body fluids.
- When you take gloves off properly, you keep the blood or fluids on the gloves from touching your skin.

Action: Taking Off Gloves

Follow these steps to take off your gloves:

Step	Action
1	Grip one glove on the *outside* of the glove near the cuff and peel it down until it comes off inside out.
2	Cup it with your other (gloved) hand.
3	Place fingers of your bare hand *inside* the cuff of the glove that is still on your hand.
4	Peel that glove off so that it comes off "inside out" with the first glove inside it.
5	If there is blood on the gloves, dispose of the gloves properly: seal them in a bag if required to do so.
6	Wash your hands after you give first aid so that you don't spread germs.

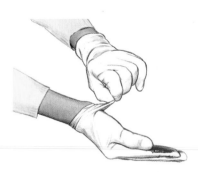

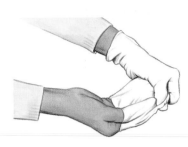

A. Grip the outside of the glove near the cuff.

B. Peel the glove down so it comes off inside out.

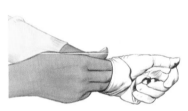

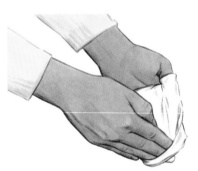

C. Place the fingers of your bare hand inside the cuff of the other glove.

D. Peel the second glove so that it comes off inside out with the first glove inside it.

Figure 3. Proper removal of protective gloves—without touching the outside of the gloves.

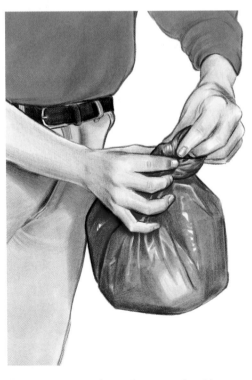

Figure 4. Dispose of waste correctly and as required by your child care center.

Definitions and Key Facts

- A first aid action plan is a written plan for a child's specific medical emergencies.
- It is a good idea for most schools, workplaces, and even families to prepare for emergencies and to make a plan for how to respond to emergencies.

Every child care facility and school should be prepared for an illness or injury emergency. A plan for such emergencies includes

- The emergency response number, which is usually 911
- The location of the first aid kit
- Instructions such as
    - Names of people in your facility who have first aid training
    - Telephone numbers and locations of nearby emergency care facilities
    - Telephone number of the poison control center

Children with illnesses may also have specific first aid action plans. For example, a child with asthma may have a specific plan explaining what to do if he has an asthma attack. (See a sample action plan, which is for a child with a seizure condition, in the Reference Materials section at the end of this workbook.)

First Aid Action Plan

Child care facilities and schools should have a health record and first aid action plan for each child who has a medical issue. A first aid action plan usually includes

- Medical history and medications
- How and when to give the medications
- Other actions to care for the ill child
- How to reach parents or guardians
- The name and telephone number of the child's healthcare provider

Make sure you know where your facility stores medications. Also make sure the medicines are stored in a way that

- Protects the privacy of the child
- Keeps them out of children's reach

The First Aid Kit

- The first aid kit should contain the supplies you'll need in the most common emergencies.
- Determine what you should keep in your kit. See the "Sample First Aid Kit" table in the Reference section for some suggestions about what you might include in your first aid kit. However, different kinds of homes or child care facilities in different parts of the country may have different needs.
- Replace what you use. If you use something in the first aid kit, replace it so that the kit is always fully supplied and ready.

Step 3: Phone 911

Definitions and Key Facts	Knowing when to phone 911 is very important in providing first aid.
What You Will Learn	You'll learn when to phone 911. You'll also learn about what you need to tell the 911 operator and what information you need to keep private.
Topics Covered	■ When to Phone for Help ■ How to Phone for Help ■ Confidentiality

When to Phone for Help

Definitions and Key Facts	The American Heart Association pediatric Chain of Survival shows some important actions needed to respond to life-threatening emergencies in children.

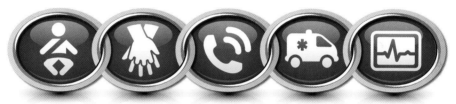

Figure 5. The AHA pediatric Chain of Survival. The first link in the pediatric chain is prevention. This is followed by early CPR, early access to emergency response services, rapid advanced life support, and integrated post-arrest care.

As a general rule, you should phone 911 and ask for help whenever

- Someone is seriously ill or injured
- You are not sure what to do in an emergency

Here are some examples of a child who is seriously ill or injured. The child

- Does not respond to voice or touch
- Has a problem breathing
- Has a severe injury
- Has a seizure
- Suddenly can't move a part of the body
- Has received an electric shock
- Has swallowed or been exposed to poison

If a child tries to commit suicide or is assaulted, phone 911 regardless of the child's condition.

Actions

- If another adult is available, ask the adult to phone 911 and get the AED and first aid kit while you stay with the child.
- If you're alone when you see or find a child who may need CPR, yell for help and send anyone who arrives to phone 911. If no one arrives, phone 911 yourself.

FYI

It's important to phone 911 before phoning anyone else. Notify parents and care-givers about any first aid you provided as soon as you are able.

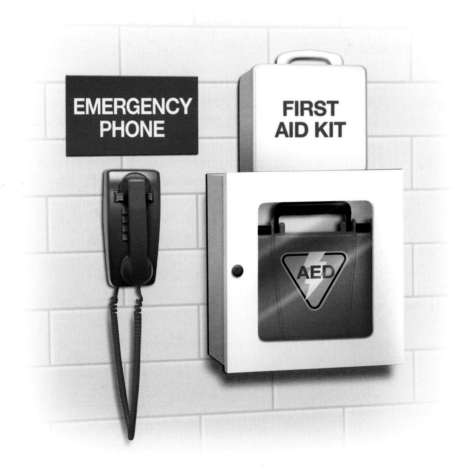

Figure 6. Know the location of the nearest phone.

How to Phone for Help

Definitions and Key Facts

Some phones inside buildings don't connect you right away to an outside line. You may have to dial 9 first to get an outside line, for example.

Your Emergency Response Number

If there is an emergency, phone _____ (fill in the blank).

Important

- Answer all of the dispatcher's questions. This is important to get help to you as fast as possible.
- Do not hang up until the dispatcher tells you to. Answering the dispatcher's questions won't delay the arrival of help.
- When you phone for help, the emergency dispatcher may be able to tell you how to do CPR, use an AED, or give first aid.
- Any time you phone 911 or provide first aid to a child, phone the child's parent or guardian as soon as possible.

Confidentiality

Definitions and Key Facts

- As a first aid rescuer, you will learn private things about children's medical conditions. Give all information about an ill or injured child only to caregivers, a healthcare provider, and anyone with more advanced training who takes over from you.
- You may also need to fill out a report. Don't share this information, except as required. Keep private things private.

Step 4: Act

Definitions and Key Facts	One of the most important parts of first aid is learning how to recognize when something is wrong.
	If a child stops acting like himself—meaning he acts differently from how he usually does—he may be sick or hurt.
	Sometimes, a child's illness or injury isn't obvious. You may only notice the child acting differently from usual. Using the Finding the Problem steps, you can often find the illness or injury.
	Once you have found the problem, you can take the next step.

What You Will Learn	You'll learn how children may act when they are sick, hurt, or abused. You'll learn steps to figure out what's wrong.

Topics Covered	■ When to Suspect Abuse
	■ How Children Act When Something Is Wrong
	■ Finding the Problem (*Skill You Will Demonstrate)

When to Suspect Abuse

Definitions and Key Facts	■ **Physical abuse:** Actions toward a child that cause bodily injuries.
	■ **Emotional abuse:** Words or actions that intentionally hurt a child emotionally or psychologically.
	– These words and actions tell children that they are worthless, unloved, unwanted, in danger, or only of value to meet someone else's needs.
	– Withholding emotional support, isolation, and terrorizing a child are forms of emotional abuse.
	■ **Sexual abuse:** Any sexual act with a child that the child is not ready for developmentally and/or can't consent to.
	■ **Neglect:** If a caregiver can provide needed care for a child and doesn't, then he is neglecting the child.
	■ Child abuse is any act that harms a child on purpose.
	■ Children of any age may be abused, and the effects of abuse can last a lifetime.
	■ Child abuse happens in every race, ethnicity, and class.
	■ Sexual abusers can be young or old, male or female, and usually are family members or acquaintances of the child.
	■ Sexual abuse by a stranger is relatively rare.

Recognizing Possible Abuse

Abused or neglected children often show signs of abuse on their bodies and in their behavior. However, children usually either cannot or will not talk about the problem.

Occasionally children will report mistreatment to an adult they trust. Take these conversations seriously and report them.

The following table lists signs of possible abuse:

• Shows sudden changes in behavior or school performance
• Has unexplained learning problems (or difficulty concentrating)
• Is always watchful, as though preparing for something bad to happen
• Is overly compliant, passive, withdrawn, or very demanding and aggressive
• Comes to school or other activities early, stays late, and does not want to go home
• Is uncomfortable with physical contact
• Has low self-esteem
• Lags in physical, emotional, or intellectual development
	• Extremely low weight for the child's age
	• Poor growth
	• Injuries that do not match the caregiver's explanation, including
	  – Bruises
	  – Broken bones
	  – Burns
	  – Bleeding, cuts, punctures
	  – Bites
	  – Blood in the diaper or underwear
	  – Trouble walking or sitting
	  – Untreated dental problems
	  – Headaches
	  – Stomachaches
	  – Poisoning
	  – Seizures
	  – Vomiting

Filing a Suspected Abuse Report

Filing an abuse report can be stressful. Reporting suspected abuse can help both the child and the family. Not reporting suspected abuse may place a child in further jeopardy, including death.

Any time you suspect child abuse, you are required to report it to law enforcement.

The identity of a person making a report is confidential and may be disclosed only by order of the court or to a law enforcement officer for investigation purposes.

Persons acting in good faith who report or assist in an investigation are usually free from civil or criminal liability.

It is important to remember that the person reporting abuse is not responsible for determining if the circumstances meet the legal definition of abuse. That is the role of law enforcement.

Shaken Baby Syndrome

Shaken baby syndrome is a kind of abuse. It happens when someone shakes an infant violently. It can severely injure the baby's eyes, neck, or brain. It can cause death.

Warning Signs of Shaken Baby Syndrome

Suspect shaken baby syndrome if an infant has some or any of the following signs and you can't figure out why. (If an infant is very cranky because he is sick or has missed his nap, don't suspect shaken baby syndrome. It's only when you can't explain the infant's behavior that you should suspect shaken baby syndrome.)

- Very sleepy or weak
- Very cranky
- Doesn't eat well or vomits for no reason
- Doesn't make sounds or smile
- Doesn't suck or swallow well
- Body gets stiff
- Has difficulty breathing
- Has seizures
- Can't lift her head
- Can't focus her eyes or follow movement

If you suspect an infant has suffered from shaken baby syndrome, phone 911.

How Children Act When Something Is Wrong

Definitions and Key Facts

- If a child acts sick or hurt, she probably is sick or hurt.
- Sick or hurt children may act younger than they are. Respond to them based on their behavior, not their age.

For detailed descriptions of what kind of behavior to expect from children of different ages, see the table "How Children Act and Tips for Interacting With Them" at the end of the First Aid section.

Action: Talking to Children

Calm and comfort a sick or hurt child. Some tips for calming a child are listed below.

- Be calm, direct, and clear.
  - Even infants will respond to your tone, if not your actual words.
  - Even toddlers who can ordinarily speak well may not be able to talk in emergencies and may bite when frustrated. If you are calm, you have the best chance to talk to and help them.
  - Adolescents may not want to talk. If you are calm, you have the best chance to talk to and help them.

- Don't talk down to children of any age.
- Kneel, squat, or get down to the child's level when you talk to him. This often helps reduce the child's fear.
- Move gently. Children might be afraid. Gentle motions may calm them.

Finding the Problem (*Skill You Will Demonstrate)

Definitions and Key Facts

- Before you can give first aid, you have to find out what the problem is. First look for problems that may be life threatening. Then look for other problems.
- **Response:** In this section, we'll talk about children responding and gasping. A child who "responds" moves, speaks, blinks, or otherwise reacts to you when you tap him and ask, "Are you OK?" A child who doesn't "respond" does nothing when you tap him and ask if he's OK.
- **Gasp:** A child who gasps usually appears to be drawing air in very quickly. He may open his mouth and move the jaw, head, or neck. Gasps may appear forceful or weak, and some time may pass between gasps since they usually happen at a slow rate. The gasp may sound like a snort, snore, or groan. Gasping is not regular or normal breathing. It is a sign of cardiac arrest in someone who doesn't respond.

Action: Finding the Problem

The following steps will help you find out what the problem is. They are listed in order of importance, with the most important step listed first.

1. When you arrive at the scene, check the scene to be sure it is safe. As you walk toward the child, look for signs of the cause of the problem.

2. Check whether the child responds. Tap the child and shout, "Are you OK?"

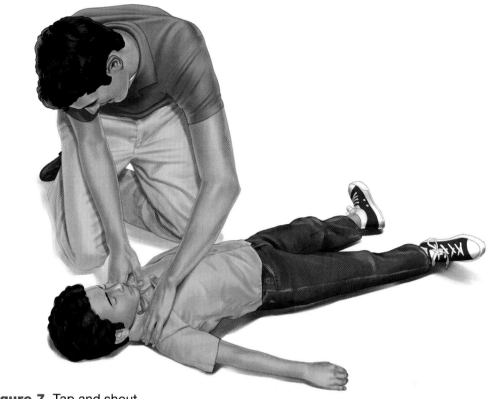

Figure 7. Tap and shout.

If the child does not respond, check if the child is breathing.

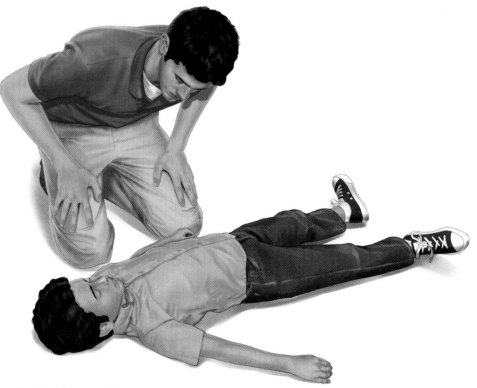

Figure 8. Check breathing.

If the child isn't breathing or is only gasping

- Begin CPR
- Send someone to phone 911 and get the first aid kit and AED

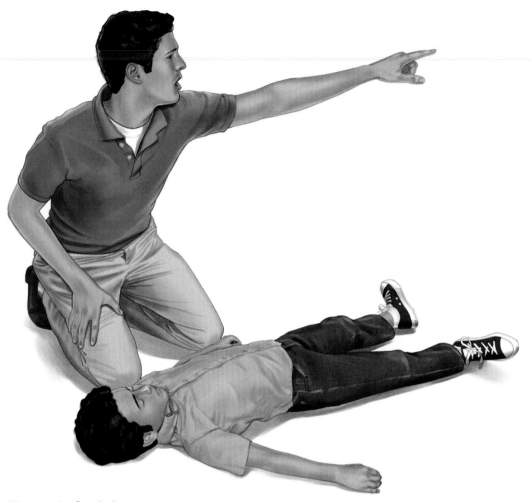

Figure 9. Get help.

If the child responds and is old enough to talk, ask what the problem is.

- A child may only be able to move, moan, or groan when you tap him and shout. If so, phone or send someone to phone 911 and get the first aid kit and AED.

3. If the child does not need CPR, look for any obvious signs of injury, such as bleeding, broken bones, burns, or bites. (You will learn about each of these problems later.)

4. Finally, look for medical information jewelry. This tells you if the child has a serious medical condition.

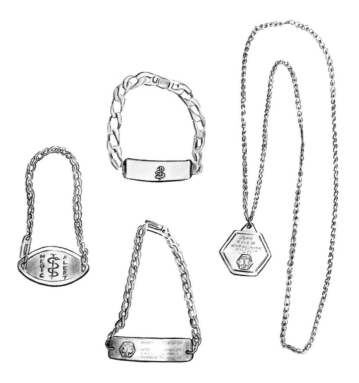

Figure 10. Medical jewelry.

Important

A child's condition may change rapidly. A child may respond and then stop responding, so check the child often.

When a child does not respond, he may stop breathing. Watch carefully to make sure that the child keeps breathing. If the child doesn't respond and is not breathing or is only gasping, give CPR.

Illnesses and Injuries

Definitions and Key Facts

You've learned what's involved in each of the 4 steps of first aid. Now, you'll learn how to put them all together in specific emergencies, from a severe allergic reaction to seizures.

Topics Covered

Group A includes illnesses and injuries you may encounter that have the potential to become serious very quickly. You'll need to act fast in these situations, because your first aid actions can make an immediate difference.

Group B includes illnesses and injuries you should be familiar with. Some may not be as urgent, but they still have the potential to become serious. One of your most important actions may be simply to recognize that something is wrong.

CPR is another way you can help. You'll learn CPR after First Aid.

Group A

Definitions and Key Facts

Group A includes illnesses and injuries you may encounter that have the potential to become serious very quickly. You'll need to act fast in these situations, because your first aid actions can make an immediate difference.

Topics Covered

- How to Stop Bleeding and Bandaging (*Skill You Will Demonstrate)
- Shock
- Mild vs Severe Allergic Reaction
- How to Use an Epinephrine Pen (*Skill You Will Demonstrate)
- Asthma
- How to Assemble and Use an Inhaler
- Dehydration
- Diabetes and Low Blood Sugar
- Heat Exhaustion
- Heat Stroke
- Hypothermia (Low Body Temperature)
- Drowning

Definitions and Key Facts

- In children, you can stop most bleeding, even bleeding that's severe, with direct pressure.
- Children often get small cuts and scrapes. However, sometimes the cut is more severe. If a child loses a lot of blood quickly, she can die. Anytime you know or suspect a child is bleeding severely, act.
- A dressing is anything you use to cover the wound and stop the bleeding.
- A dressing can be a gauze pad or any other clean piece of cloth or even a gloved hand.
- Dressings help prevent infection.
- A bandage is material used to protect or cover an injured body part.
- A bandage may also help keep pressure on the wound.

Step 1: Prevent

- Use the Child and Infant Safety Checklist to help keep a child safe.
- Use dressings to help prevent infection.
- Use antibiotic cream on small scrapes and surface cuts to prevent infection. (Make sure the child doesn't have an allergy to antibiotic cream first.)

Step 2: Be Safe

- Make sure the scene is safe.
- Get the first aid kit.
- Wear PPE.
- If the injured child can help you, ask him to put direct pressure on the wound while you put on your PPE.

Step 3: Phone 911

Phone 911

- If there is a lot of bleeding (severe bleeding)
- If you cannot stop the bleeding
- If you suspect a head, neck, or spine injury
- If you are not sure what to do
- If you see signs of shock. Signs of shock include
  - Feeling weak, faint, or dizzy
  - Being nauseous
  - Breathing very fast
  - Acting restless, confused, or unusually sleepy
  - Looking pale
  - Being cold to the touch

Step 4: Act   Follow these steps to stop bleeding:

Step	Action
1	Find the place that's bleeding.
2	If the cut or scrape is minor, wash the area with lots of clean water and soap if available to get the wound clean before applying the dressings.
3	Put a dressing on the wound.
4	Apply direct pressure on the dressing. Use the flat part of your fingers or the palm of your hand.
5	If the bleeding does not stop, add more dressings on top of the first and press harder.
6	Keep pressure on the wound until it stops bleeding.
7	If you can't keep pressure on the wound, wrap a bandage firmly over the dressing to hold the dressing in place and to keep pressure on the wound.

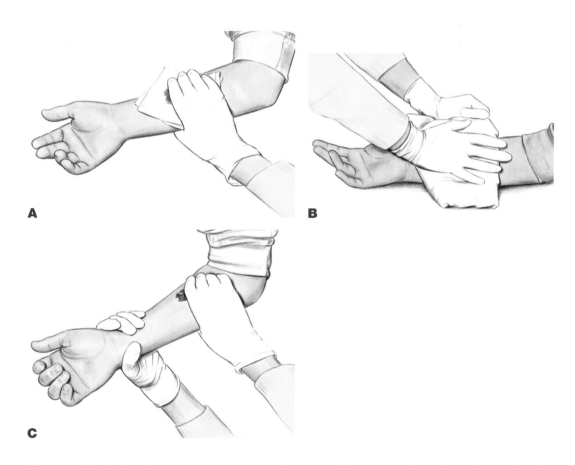

Figure 11. A dressing can be a gauze pad or pads (**A**) or any other clean piece of cloth (**B**). If you do not have a dressing, use your gloved hand (**C**).

■ You'll use less direct pressure to stop the bleeding for a minor cut or scrape than for a major cut or scrape.

■ Use antibiotic cream on small scrapes and surface cuts to prevent infection. (Make sure the child doesn't have an allergy to antibiotic cream first.)

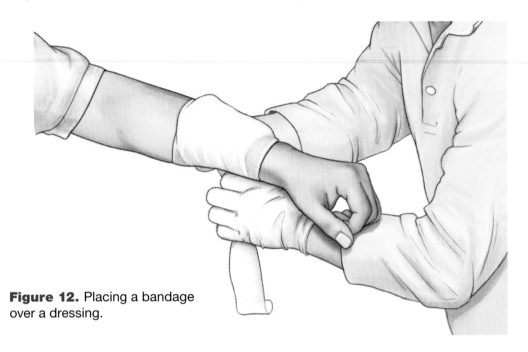

Figure 12. Placing a bandage over a dressing.

FYI

■ If a nosebleed doesn't stop after about 15 minutes, or if the child has trouble breathing, phone 911.

■ If you can stop the bleeding with direct pressure, you may need only a small bandage or no bandage at all.

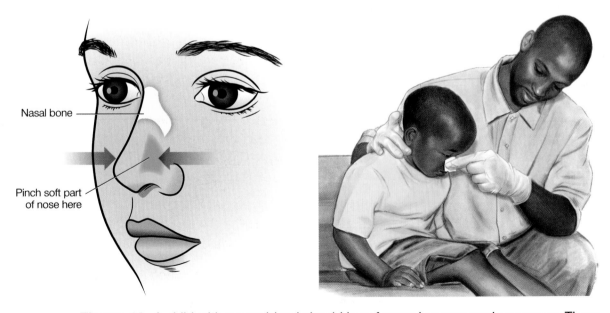

Nasal bone

Pinch soft part of nose here

Figure 13. A child with a nosebleed should lean forward as you apply pressure. There are several common myths about stopping nosebleeds. Be sure the child leans forward and that you pinch the soft part of the nose.

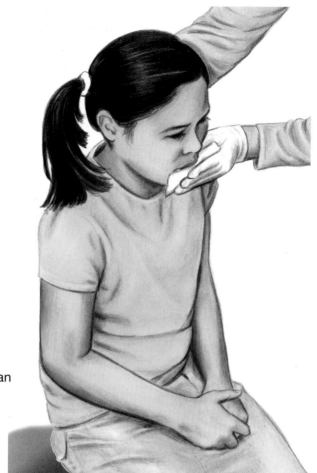

Figure 14. If the child has a mouth injury, watch for trouble breathing. Sometimes bleeding in the mouth can block the airway.

Shock

Definitions and Key Facts

- Sometimes the inside of the body is injured. The skin may not be broken, so there may not be any blood you can see, but something (an organ, a blood vessel) beneath the skin is hurt and is bleeding inside the body. This kind of blood loss is serious and can lead to shock.

- There are different kinds of shock. One of the most common happens when a child has lost too much blood or water.

- A child may lose a lot of fluid in a short period of time. This child may still look somewhat normal for a short while.

- Shock can be fatal.

- Shock isn't an illness a child can just "get." Another illness or injury always causes it. One common cause of shock is bleeding inside the body.

Watch for shock especially if a child is not acting like himself and

- Has recently lost fluid, such as with vomiting or diarrhea, and has a fever
- Loses a lot of blood, including bleeding inside the body
- Has a severe allergic reaction

Suspect bleeding inside the body if a child has

- An injury from a car crash, from being hit by a car, or after a fall from a height
- An injury to the abdomen or chest (including bruises caused by seat belt marks)
- Sports injuries such as slamming into other people or being hit with a ball
- Pain in the chest or abdomen after an injury
- Shortness of breath after an injury
- Coughed-up or vomited blood after an injury
- Signs of shock without bleeding that you can see
- A knife or gunshot wound

Step 1: Prevent

Use the Child and Infant Safety Checklist to help prevent injuries that lead to severe bleeding.

Step 2: Be Safe

- Make sure the scene is safe.
- Get the first aid kit.
- Wear PPE.

Step 3: Phone 911

Phone 911

- If there is a lot of bleeding (severe bleeding)
- If you cannot stop the bleeding
- If you see signs of shock (listed in the following action table)

Step 4: Act

Follow these steps to help a child in shock:

Step	Action
1	A child in shock doesn't act like himself. Signs of shock include • Feeling weak, faint, or dizzy • Being nauseous • Breathing very fast • Acting restless, confused, or unusually sleepy • Looking pale • Being cold to the touch
2	Help the child lie on her back.
3	Use pressure to stop any bleeding you can see.
4	Cover the child to keep the child warm (you can use a blanket if there is one in the first aid kit).

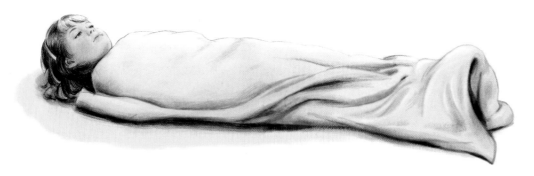

Figure 15. Cover a child in shock.

Mild vs Severe Allergic Reaction

Definitions and Key Facts

Many allergic reactions are mild. Some reactions that seem mild can become severe within minutes.

Step 1: Prevent

Children can be allergic to many things, including

- Many foods, such as eggs, nuts, chocolate
- Insect stings or bites, especially bee or wasp stings

Step 2: Be Safe

- Make sure the scene is safe.
- Get the first aid kit.
- Wear PPE.

Step 3: Phone 911

Phone 911

- If the allergy is severe

Step 4: Act

Figure out if an allergic reaction is mild or severe:

Mild Allergic Reaction	Severe Allergic Reaction

• A stuffy nose, sneezing, and itching around the eyes
• Itching of the skin
• Raised, red rash on the skin
	• The child may have some mild symptoms and also 1 or more of the following:
	  – Trouble breathing
	  – Swelling of the tongue and face
	  – Fainting

If the reaction is severe, you may need to use the child's epinephrine pen, in addition to phoning 911.

Definitions and Key Facts

- An epinephrine pen will help a child with a severe allergic reaction breathe more easily. It contains a small amount of medicine that can be injected through clothing.
- Some states and organizations permit first aid rescuers to help people use their epinephrine pens. People who carry epinephrine pens usually know when and how to use them.
- You may help give the injection if you are approved to do so by your state regulations and by your child care center.
- It usually takes several minutes before the medicine starts to work. The epinephrine injection is given in the side of the thigh.
- There are 2 doses of epinephrine pens, 1 for adults and 1 for children. Make sure you have the epinephrine pen prescribed for that child. If the child can't use the pen himself, and if you are allowed to, give him an injection.

Afterward, be sure to dispose of the pen properly or give it to someone with more advanced training, so that no one is accidentally stuck by the needle.

Step 1: Prevent

People can be allergic to many things, including

- Many foods, such as eggs, nuts, chocolate
- Insect stings or bites, especially bee or wasp stings

Step 2: Be Safe

- Make sure the scene is safe.
- Get the first aid kit.
- Wear PPE.

Step 3: Phone 911

Phone 911

- If the allergy is severe

Step 4: Act

Follow these steps to use an epinephrine pen:

Step	Action
1	Figure out if the allergic reaction is mild or severe. If it is severe, go to step 2.
2	Get the child's prescribed epinephrine pen.
3	Take off the safety cap. Follow the instructions on the pen.
4	Hold the epinephrine pen in your fist without touching either end, because the needle comes out of one end.

(continued)

(continued)

Step	Action
5	Press the tip of the pen hard against the side of the child's thigh, about halfway between the hip and knee. Give the injection through clothes or on bare skin.
6	Hold the pen in place for about 10 seconds.
7	Remove the needle by pulling the pen straight out.

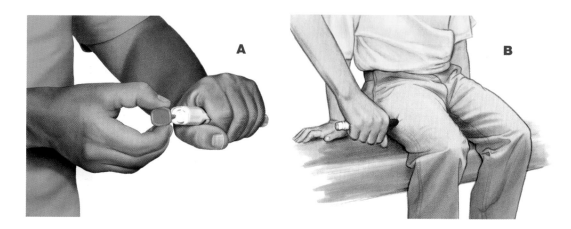

Figure 16. A, Take off the safety cap. **B,** Use the pen.

FYI

It's important to dispose of needles correctly so that no one gets stuck accidentally. Your center may have a policy about the best way to dispose of needles and other "sharps." If you are not sure what to do, ask someone with more advanced training.

Asthma

Definitions and Key Facts

- Asthma is common in children. It is a disease of the air passages. Air passages carry air to the lungs.
- Some children with asthma must take daily medication. Others take medicine only when they have asthma symptoms. Many children with asthma have an inhaler.
- A spacer is a tool that fits on an inhaler and helps deliver the medicine more efficiently.
- Your child care center or school should have a first aid action plan for every child with asthma.
- If a child has an asthma attack, send another adult for the plan and the child's medicines.

Step 1: Prevent Help the child avoid things that trigger his asthma, such as cold air and cigarette smoke.

Step 2: Be Safe
- Make sure the scene is safe.
- Get the first aid kit.
- Wear PPE.

Step 3: Phone 911 Phone 911
- If a child with asthma has trouble breathing, even after taking medication

Step 4: Act Follow these steps to help a child who is having an asthma attack:

Step	Action
1	During an asthma attack, a child may have • Trouble breathing • Coughing • Tightness in the chest • Wheezing (whistling sound) • Fast breathing
2	Keep calm and soothe the child. Crying can make the asthma attack worse.
3	If the child has a prescription for asthma medicine, get the medicine and help the child take it.
4	Check the child's breathing. If the child is having trouble breathing, phone 911.
5	Be prepared to start CPR if the child stops responding and stops breathing.
6	Stay with the child until someone with more training arrives and takes over.

How to Assemble and Use an Inhaler

Definitions and Key Facts
- Many children with medical conditions, such as asthma, know about their conditions and carry inhaler medicine.
- The medicine can make them feel better within minutes of using it.
- Sometimes children have so much trouble breathing, they need help using their inhalers.

Step 1: Prevent
If a child in your care has an inhaler, make an action plan with the parent or guardian for how and when to use it.

Step 2: Be Safe
Make sure the scene is safe.

Step 3: Phone 911
Phone 911

- If the child has no medicine
- If the child does not get better after using her medicine
- If the child's breathing gets worse, the child has trouble speaking, or the child stops responding

Step 4: Act

- When someone has trouble breathing, she may panic.
- Younger children may not be able to use their inhalers at all.
- You may need to assemble the inhaler and help a child use it.

Inhalers are made up of 2 parts: the medicine canister and the mouthpiece. A spacer can be attached that makes it easier for the child with the breathing problem to inhale all the medicine.

Follow these steps to assemble and use an inhaler:

Step	Action
1	Shake the medicine.
2	Put the medicine canister into the mouthpiece.
3	Remove the cap from the mouthpiece.
4	Attach a spacer if there is one available and if you know how.
5	Tilt the child's head back slightly and have him breathe out slowly.
6	Put the inhaler or spacer in the child's mouth.
7	Push down on the top of the medicine canister. Have the child breathe in slowly and deeply as you push down.
8	Have the child hold his breath for 10 seconds and then breathe out slowly.

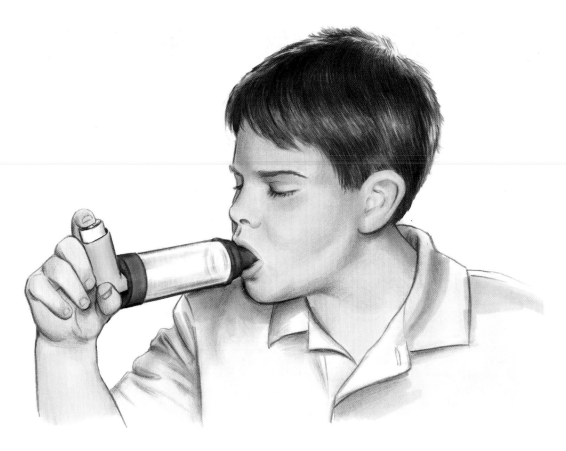

Figure 17. Using an inhaler with a spacer.

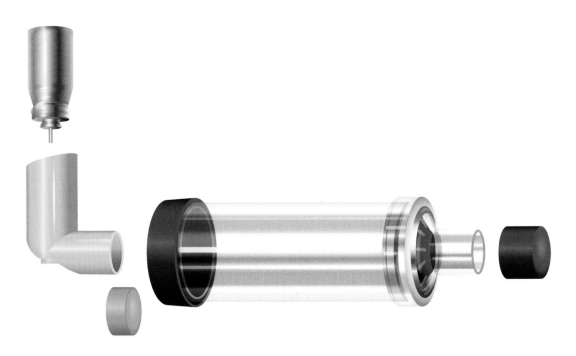

Figure 18. The parts of an inhaler: medicine canister, mouthpiece, and spacer.

Dehydration

Definitions and Key Facts

- A child gets dehydrated when she doesn't have enough fluid in her body.
- This often happens when a child loses a lot of fluid through vomiting or diarrhea and doesn't drink enough to replace the fluid she has lost.
- Dehydration is included in the section on life-threatening illnesses because while it is rarely fatal in itself, it can lead to shock, which can be fatal.
- If you watch for and help with dehydration, you can help avoid shock.
- It can take a little while for a sick child's body to lose enough fluid to go into shock.

Step 1: Prevent

- If you help a dehydrated child, you can help prevent shock.
- Make sure a child drinks and eats enough to stay hydrated.

Step 2: Be Safe

- Make sure the scene is safe.
- Get the first aid kit.
- Wear PPE.

Step 3: Phone 911

Phone 911

- If you see signs of shock

Step 4: Act

Follow these steps for dehydration:

Step	Action
1	Watch for dehydration if • The child vomits, has diarrhea, or has fever for 12 or more hours • The child drinks less than usual
2	Signs of dehydration include • Weakness • Thirst • Dry mouth • Less urination than usual • Less hunger than usual
3	If you suspect a child is dehydrated, contact a healthcare provider right away.

Diabetes and Low Blood Sugar

Definitions and Key Facts

Some diabetics take insulin to control their blood sugar. Too much insulin can cause low blood sugar.

Children with diabetes who are not acting normally may have an illness or injury that is unrelated to diabetes. Be sure to check the child for other illnesses and injuries.

Low blood sugar can occur if a child with diabetes has

- Not eaten or is vomiting
- Not eaten enough food for the level of activity
- Injected too much insulin

Step 1: Prevent

A child with diabetes has probably received specific instruction from a health-care provider on how to maintain his health. Some of the ways a child with diabetes can prevent low blood sugar include

- Keeping track of the amount of sugar in his blood
- Following a diet designed for children with diabetes
- Following his doctor's directions for taking his insulin

Step 2: Be Safe

- Make sure the scene is safe.
- Get the first aid kit.
- Wear PPE.

Step 3: Phone 911

Phone 911

- If the child does not feel better within a few minutes after eating or drinking something containing sugar
- If you check the sugar and it is not low but the child is still not acting normally

Step 4: Act

Follow these steps to help a child with low blood sugar:

Step	Action
1	Signs of low blood sugar can appear quickly and may include • A change in behavior, such as confusion or irritability • Sleepiness or even not responding • Hunger, thirst, or weakness • Sweating, pale skin color • A seizure (see the section on seizures)
2	Check the child's first aid action plan. Follow the plan, including directions about how to check blood sugar.
3	If you suspect or have confirmed that the blood sugar is low and the child can sit up and swallow, give the child something containing sugar to eat or drink.
4	Have the child sit quietly or lie down.

FYI: What to Give for Low Blood Sugar

It's important to make sure that whatever you give has sugar in it. Diet foods and drinks don't have sugar; chocolate doesn't have enough sugar. For a child with diabetes who has low blood sugar, give

- Fruit juice
- Sugar
- Regular soft drink
- Whatever the parent or guardian instructs you to give to the child

Important

If a child with low blood sugar is unable to sit up and swallow, don't give him anything to eat or drink.

FYI: Diabetic Emergency Supplies

Children with diabetes often have emergency supplies in case of low blood sugar. Make sure the first aid action plan says where the supplies are and that you can get to them quickly in an emergency.

If you are a child care worker or teacher and have a child with diabetes in your care, make an action plan with the child's parent or guardian.

Heat Exhaustion

Definitions and Key Facts

- Most heat-related emergencies are caused by vigorous exercise in a warm or hot environment.
- Infants and children have more trouble keeping their bodies at the right temperature than adults.

- Heat exhaustion is included in this section because while heat exhaustion is not life threatening, it can quickly turn into heat stroke, which is life threatening. It often occurs when someone exercises in the heat and sweats a lot.

Step 1: Prevent

- Children should stay hydrated before exercise.
- Drinking often—water or sports drinks—helps a child stay hydrated during exercise.
- Children should wear lightweight clothes in light colors when exercising in the sun or heat.
- If it's hot or humid, children ideally should avoid exercising outdoors.
- Children should exercise during cooler times of the day.
- Carefully watch children who aren't fit or aren't used to exercising in the heat.
- If a child looks sick or not normal/not like himself, have him stop exercising and check for heat exhaustion or heat stroke.

Step 2: Be Safe

- Make sure the scene is safe.
- Get the first aid kit.
- Wear PPE.

Step 3: Phone 911

Phone 911

- If you suspect heat exhaustion.

Step 4: Act

Follow these steps to help a child with heat exhaustion:

Step	Action
1	Look for the following signs of heat exhaustion: • Sweating • Nausea • Dizziness • Vomiting • Muscle cramps • Feeling faint • Fatigue If you suspect the child has heat exhaustion, begin the rest of the steps right away.
2	Have the child lie down in a cool place.
3	Remove as much of the child's clothing as possible.
4	Cool the child with a cool water spray.
5	If cool water spray is not available, place cool damp cloths on the neck, armpit, and groin area.
6	Have the child drink something that contains sugar and electrolytes, such as juice or a sports drink, or water if the others aren't available.

Heat Stroke

Definitions and Key Facts

- Heat stroke is a very serious condition.
- It looks similar to heat exhaustion, but it is life threatening.
- Act quickly.

Step 1: Prevent

- Follow the same prevention steps you would for heat exhaustion.
- Helping a child who has heat exhaustion will help prevent heat exhaustion from becoming heat stroke.
- Never leave a child or infant in a hot car.

Step 2: Be Safe

- Make sure the scene is safe.
- Get the first aid kit.
- Wear PPE.
- Get the AED.

Step 3: Phone 911

Phone 911

- If you suspect heat stroke

Step 4: Act

Follow these steps to help a child with heat stroke:

Step	Action
1	Look for the following signs of heat stroke: Key signs of heat stroke are • Confusion • Passing out • Dizziness • Seizures Other signs of heat stroke include • Nausea • Vomiting • Muscle cramps • Feeling faint • Fatigue If you suspect the child has heat stroke, begin the rest of the steps right away.
2	Put the child in cool water, up to her neck if possible.
3	If you can't put the child in cool water up to her neck, go through the steps for heat exhaustion.
4	See if the child needs CPR.

Hypothermia (Low Body Temperature)

Definitions and Key Facts

- Cold injury to the whole body is called low body temperature, or hypothermia.
- Hypothermia occurs when body temperature falls. Hypothermia is a serious condition that can cause death.
- A child can develop hypothermia even when the temperature is above freezing. For example, a child could get hypothermia from walking in rain and wind without a jacket.
- Infants and very small children can easily develop hypothermia.
- Shivering protects the body by producing heat. Shivering stops when the body becomes very cold.

Step 1: Prevent

- Make sure children wear appropriate clothing in cold weather.
- Watch small children closely if they are in very cold weather to make sure they stay warm.

Step 2: Be Safe

- Make sure the scene is safe.
- Get the first aid kit and AED.
- Wear PPE.

Step 3: Phone 911

Phone 911

- If you suspect hypothermia

Step 4: Act

Follow these steps to help a child with hypothermia:

Step	Action
1	Look for signs of hypothermia, which include the following: • The skin is cool to the touch. • The child is shivering (shivering stops when the body temperature is very low). • The child may become confused or drowsy. • Personality may change or the child may behave as if unconcerned about the condition. • Muscles become stiff and rigid, and the skin becomes ice-cold and blue. As the body temperature continues to drop • The child stops responding • The child's breathing slows • It may be hard to tell whether the child is breathing • The child may appear dead
2	Get the child out of the cold.
3	See if the child needs CPR.
4	Remove wet clothing and pat the body dry. Put dry clothes on the child and cover her with a blanket.

(continued)

Step	Action
5	Wrap the child up with anything you have—clothing, towels, newspapers, etc. Cover the head but not the face.

Drowning

Definitions and Key Facts

- Drowning is the third most common accidental cause of death in children under 15 years of age.
- Children are very attracted to water. Young children can drown in very shallow water, for instance, a 5-gallon bucket or even in the bathtub.

Step 1: Prevent

- Do not leave a child alone around any water.
  - The head of an infant or a small child is very heavy compared with the rest of his body.
  - Infants and small children can lean and fall into a bucket, toilet, or small container and be unable to lift their heads out of the water.
- Swimming pools, creeks, fountains, lakes, and rivers are very interesting to most children. It is important to closely watch all children near pools or other bodies of water.
  - Any infant or child can drown, even if the child knows how to swim.
  - Always stay within reach of a child near a body of water.
  - Use life jackets when appropriate.

Step 2: Be Safe

- Make sure that the scene is safe for you and the child.
- Get the first aid kit.

Step 3: Phone 911

Phone 911:

- Always phone 911 in case of drowning.

Step 4: Act

If you see a child who may be drowning, follow these steps:

Step	Action
1	If the child is under water, get her out safely.
2	Check if the child needs CPR. If she does, give it.
3	If the child doesn't need CPR, remove wet clothing and wrap the child in dry blankets. Continue to check if the child needs CPR.

FYI: Drowning in Cold Water

Children who drown in cold water may appear dead: they may have stiff muscles; they may not be breathing; and their skin may be cold and blue. Start CPR right away and continue until someone with more advanced training arrives and takes over.

49

Group B

Amputations

Definitions and Key Facts

- If a part of the body, such as a finger, toe, hand, or foot, is cut off (amputated), save the body part because doctors may be able to reattach it.
- You can preserve a detached body part at room temperature, but it will be in better condition to be reattached if you keep it cool.

Step 1: Prevent

Use the Child and Infant Safety Checklist to create a safer environment.

Step 2: Be Safe

- Make sure the scene is safe.
- Get the first aid kit.
- Wear PPE.

Step 3: Phone 911

Phone 911

- If a body part is amputated

Step 4: Act

Follow these steps when a part of the body has been amputated:

Step	Action
1	Find the part of the body that has been amputated.
2	Stop the bleeding with firm pressure.
3	If you find the amputated part, protect it. To protect an amputated part • Rinse it with clean water. • Cover or wrap it with a clean dressing. • If it will fit, place it in a watertight plastic bag. • Place that bag in another container with ice or ice and water. • Label the bag with the child's name, date, and time. • Send it to the hospital with the child.
4	Keep the child still until someone with more training arrives.

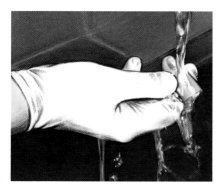
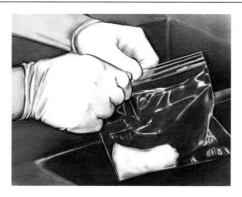
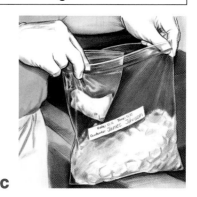

A   B   C

Figure 19. Protect the amputated part. **A,** If you can find the amputated part, rinse it with clean water. **B,** If it will fit, place the wrapped part in a watertight plastic bag. **C,** Place that bag in another labeled bag.

Important

Always put something in between a body part and the ice and water. Direct contact with ice or ice and water may damage the body part.

Bites and Stings

The main actions you can take for a bite or sting are to
- Wash the bite or sting area well with lots of running water and soap if available
- Put a bag of ice and water on the bite
- Watch for allergic reactions
- Check if the child needs CPR (particularly after a poisonous bite)

The action tables offer specific steps for different bites and stings, including
- Human and animal bites
- Snakebites
- Insect and bee stings and bites
- Marine bites and stings
- Ticks

Definitions and Key Facts	■ Young, preschool-aged children sometimes bite each other. Some young children will bite others to show their feelings.
	■ Most children stop biting when they grow older.
	■ Animal bites are less common and can often be prevented. Unfortunately, when they do occur, animal bites can be serious.
	■ When a bite breaks the skin, the wound can bleed and may become infected from the germs in the child's or animal's mouth. Bites that do not break the skin usually are not serious.

Step 1: Prevent
- Some bites get infected. You can help prevent this by washing small wounds well as soon as possible.
- Teach children how to safely approach dogs they are not familiar with (calmly, slowly, check with the owner first before approaching or petting).

Step 2: Be Safe
- Make sure the scene is safe.
- Stay away from any animal that acts strangely.
- Get the first aid kit.
- Wear PPE.

Step 3: Phone 911

Phone 911
- If the child has been bitten by an animal

Step 4: Act

Follow these steps to help a child with a human or animal bite:

Step	Action
1	Find where the child was bitten.
2	Wash the wound with a lot of running water (and soap if available).
3	Stop any bleeding with pressure and bandages.
4	For all bites that break the skin, phone a healthcare provider.
5	If there is a bruise or swelling, place a bag of ice and water wrapped in a towel on the bite for up to 20 minutes.

Important
- These animals may carry rabies: cat, dog, skunk, raccoon, fox, bat, or other wild animal.
- If a child has been alone in a room with a bat, contact a healthcare provider.

Definitions and Key Facts	▪ If you recognize the type of snake, tell the people with more advanced training what kind of snake bit the child.
	▪ If you aren't sure whether a snake is poisonous, assume it is.

Step 1: Prevent

▪ Teach children to leave snakes alone, stay away from snakes, and tell an adult when they come across a snake.

▪ Keep outdoor play areas away from places where snakes can live, including piles of rock or firewood, as well as tall grass.

▪ Teach children not to reach into areas where they can't see what may be hidden.

Step 2: Be Safe

▪ Make sure the scene is safe.

▪ Be very careful around a wounded snake.

▪ Back away and go around the snake.

▪ If a snake has been hurt or killed, leave it alone. A snake might bite even when severely hurt or close to death.

▪ If a snake needs to be moved, use a long-handled shovel. If you don't need to move it, leave it alone.

▪ Get the first aid kit.

▪ Wear PPE.

Step 3: Phone 911

Phone 911

▪ If the child has been bitten by a snake

Step 4: Act

Follow these steps to help a child with a snakebite:

Step	Action
1	Look for signs of a poisonous snakebite. They are • Pain in the bite area that keeps getting worse • Swelling of the bite area • Nausea, vomiting, sweating, and weakness
2	Ask another adult to move any other people inside or away from the area.
3	Tell the bitten child to be still and calm. Tell him to avoid moving the part of the body that was bitten.
4	Remove any tight clothing and jewelry.
5	Gently wash the bite area with running water (and soap, if available).

Important	Some people have heard about other ways to provide first aid for a snakebite, such as sucking out poison. The correct steps are in the table.

Insect and Bee Stings and Bites

Definitions and Key Facts	Usually, insect and spider bites and stings cause only mild pain, itching, and swelling at the bite. Some insect bites can be serious and even fatal if ■ The child bitten has a severe allergic reaction to the bite or sting ■ Poison (venom) is injected into the child (for example, from a black widow spider or brown recluse spider)
Step 1: Prevent	■ Keep children from bothering insects. ■ Use insect repellent that is approved for use on children. ■ If you know a child has a severe allergy to an insect or bee sting, keep his prescribed epinephrine pen close by at all times. ■ Have children wear light-colored clothing that covers the arms and legs when walking or playing in areas where flying insects are likely to be. ■ Keep flowering plants and gardens far from where children play. ■ Put outdoor toys away so spiders and insects can't hide inside them.
Step 2: Be Safe	■ Make sure the scene is safe. ■ Get the first aid kit. ■ Wear PPE.
Step 3: Phone 911	Phone 911 ■ If the child has signs of a severe allergic reaction ■ If the child tells you that she has a severe allergic reaction to insect bites or stings ■ If the child needs CPR

Step 4: Act

Follow these steps to give first aid to a child with an insect or spider bite or sting:

Step	Action
1	If the child has a severe allergic reaction to insect bites or stings and has an epinephrine pen, get the pen.
2	If a **bee** stung the child: • Look for the stinger. Bees are the only insects that may leave their stingers behind. • Scrape away the stinger and venom sac using something with a dull edge such as a credit card.
3	**Wash** the bite or sting area with a **lot of running water** (and soap, if possible).
4	Put a **bag of ice and water** wrapped in a towel or cloth over the bite or sting area for up to 20 minutes.
5	See if the child needs CPR. If so, give CPR.
6	Watch the child for at least 30 minutes for signs of an allergic reaction.

Important

The following are the signs of poisonous spider and scorpion bites and stings. Some of the signs may vary depending on the type of bite or sting. If you see any of these signs, follow the action table above.

- Severe pain at the site of the bite or sting
- Muscle cramps
- Headache
- Fever
- Vomiting
- Seizures
- Lack of response

FYI

With bee stings, make sure you remove the stinger with something flat and dull that won't squeeze the stinger. Squeezing the venom sac can release more venom (poison).

Definitions and Key Facts	Marine fish and animals can bite or sting humans.

- This happens most often in salt water.
- The bites and stings may cause pain, swelling, redness, or bleeding.
- They may also cause infection or an allergic reaction.

Some marine bites and stings can be serious and even fatal if

- The bitten child has a severe allergic reaction to the bite or sting
- Poison (venom) is injected into the child (for example, from a jellyfish, stingray, or stonefish)

Step 1: Prevent

- Use the Child and Infant Safety Checklist to help keep a child safe.
- At the beach, pay attention to signs that warn you about dangerous jellyfish or other marine life.
  - Even dead marine animals can sting you.
  - Avoid touching them with bare hands or skin.

Step 2: Be Safe

- Make sure the scene is safe.
- Get the first aid kit.
- Wear PPE. Always use something to protect your bare skin from touching a biting or stinging marine animal.
- Even if you are wearing PPE, try to avoid touching a biting or stinging marine animal.

Step 3: Phone 911

Phone 911

- If a child has been bitten or stung by a marine animal and has signs of a severe allergic reaction
- If a child was bitten or stung in an area known to have poisonous marine animals

Step 4: Act

Follow these steps to help a child with a marine bite or sting:

Step	Action
1	The following are signs of a poisonous marine bite or sting: • Chest pain • Cramps • Fever • Weakness, faintness, or dizziness • Nausea or vomiting • Numbness or trouble moving parts of the body • Severe pain, swelling, or discoloration of area bitten or stung
2	Keep the child quiet and still.
3	Wipe off stingers or tentacles with a gloved hand or towel.
4	Wash off remaining marine animal parts with salt (ocean) water.
5	If the sting is from a jellyfish, rinse the injured area for at least 30 seconds with lots of vinegar. Then put the part of the body that was stung in hot water. You may also have the child take a shower with water as hot as he can bear, for at least 20 minutes, or as long as pain persists.

FYI

- For all bites and stings that break the skin, see a healthcare provider.
- On jellyfish stings, if vinegar is not available, use a baking soda and water solution instead.
- On jellyfish stings, if hot water is not available, apply dry hot or cold packs for up to 20 minutes instead.

Ticks

Definitions and Key Facts

- Ticks are found on animals and in wooded areas. They attach themselves to exposed body parts. Many ticks are harmless. Some carry serious diseases.
- If you find a tick, remove it as soon as possible. The longer the tick stays attached to a child, the greater the child's chance of catching a disease.

Step 1: Prevent

- Children should wear light-colored clothing so you can see the tick more easily later.
- Clothing should cover a child's arms and legs. Tuck pants into the child's socks or boots.
- Children should avoid wooded or brushy areas with high grass and leaf litter.
- Children should walk in the center of trails.
- Use repellants that contain no more than 30% DEET for children over 2 months of age as long as the label says it is safe for use on children.

- Use DEET products only on infants older than 2 months.
- Do not use sunscreen with DEET because of the need to reapply sunscreen frequently.

Step 2: Be Safe
- Make sure the scene is safe.
- Get the first aid kit.
- Wear PPE.

Step 3: Phone 911

Usually, you do not need to phone 911 for a tick bite.

Step 4: Act

Follow these steps to help a child with a tick bite:

Step	Action
1	Find the tick.
2	Grab the tick by its mouth or head as close to the skin as possible with tweezers or a tick-removing device.
3	Lift the tick straight out without twisting or squeezing its body.
4	Wash the bite with running water (and soap, if available).
5	See a healthcare provider if you are in an area where tick-borne diseases occur. If possible, place the tick in a plastic bag and give it to the healthcare provider.

Important
- If you lift the tick until the child's skin tents and wait for several seconds, the tick may let go.
- Some people have heard about other ways to remove a tick. The correct way to remove a tick is to follow the actions in the table.

Broken Bones, Sprains, and Bruises

Definitions and Key Facts
- Joint sprains happen when joints move in directions they're not supposed to.
- Without an x-ray, it may be impossible to tell whether a bone is broken, but you will perform the same actions even if you don't know whether the bone is broken.
- A child may get a bruise if he is hit or runs into a hard object. Bruises happen when blood collects under the skin. They can appear as red or black-and-blue spots.

Step 1: Prevent

Use the Child and Infant Safety Checklist to help keep a child safe.

Step 2: Be Safe
- Make sure the scene is safe.
- Get the first aid kit.
- Wear PPE.

Step 3: Phone 911

Phone 911

- If there is a large open wound
- If the injured part is abnormally bent
- If you're not sure what to do

Step 4: Act

Follow these steps to help a child with bruises, broken bones, or sprains:

Step	Action
1	Look for broken bones or sprains. The signs include • Swelling • Pain • Not being able to move the injured part • A joint turning slightly blue
2	Cover any open wound with a clean dressing.
3	Put a plastic bag filled with ice and water on the injured area with a towel between the ice bag and the skin for up to 20 minutes.
4	If an injured body part hurts, the child should avoid using it until checked by a healthcare provider.

You can use a bag of frozen vegetables if ice is not available. You may use a cold pack, but it is not as cold and may not work as well as ice and water.

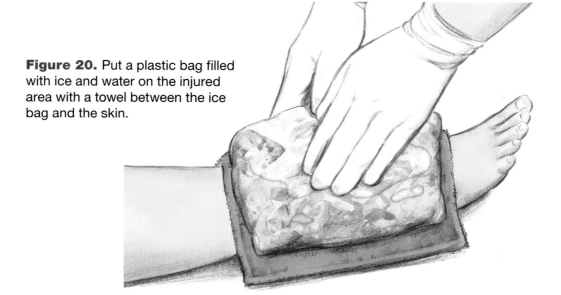

Figure 20. Put a plastic bag filled with ice and water on the injured area with a towel between the ice bag and the skin.

Remove jewelry from the injured area if possible.

Splinting

Definitions and Key Facts	▪ A splint keeps an injured body part from moving. In general, healthcare providers apply splints. ▪ At times, you may need to splint an arm or a leg. For example, if you are hiking in the wilderness, you may need to splint an injured arm. ▪ Rolled-up towels, magazines, and pieces of wood can be used as splints.
Step 1: Prevent	Use the Child and Infant Safety Checklist to help keep a child safe.
Step 2: Be Safe	▪ Make sure the scene is safe. ▪ Get the first aid kit. ▪ Wear PPE.
Step 3: Phone 911	Phone 911 ▪ If there is a large open wound ▪ If the injured part is abnormally bent ▪ If you're not sure what to do

Step 4: Act

Follow these steps to splint an injured body part to protect it and keep it still:

Step	Action
1	To make a splint, use something (such as a magazine) that will keep the arm or leg from moving.
2	Ideally, place the splint so that it extends beyond the injured area and supports the joints above and below the injury.
3	Tie the splint to the injured body part so that it supports the injured area. Use tape, gauze, or cloth to secure it.
4	Make sure the child is checked by a healthcare provider.

FYI

▪ You should be able to put a few fingers between the splint and the injured body part. Do not tie the splint too tightly or straighten an injured body part. This might cause more pain or injury.

▪ If you use something hard for the splint, pad the inside of the splint with cloths or dressings, if possible, to keep the child comfortable.

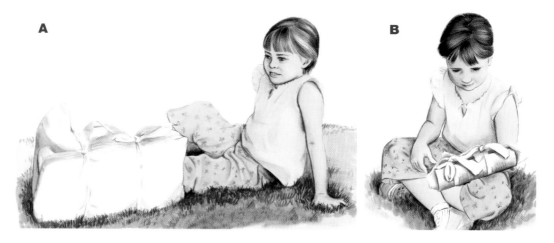

A

B

Figure 21. A splint keeps an injured body part from moving.

Burns and Electrical Injuries

Burns

Definitions and Key Facts

- Burns are injuries that can be caused by contact with heat, electricity, or chemicals. Heat burns can be caused by contact with fire, a hot surface, a hot liquid, or steam.
- Use cold water on burns. Ice can damage burned areas. If someone with a burn gets too cold, she can get hypothermia (low body temperature).

Step 1: Prevent

- Keep hot foods and drinks out of children's reach.
- Make sure food isn't too hot before feeding it to children, especially infants.
- When using small heating appliances, such as irons, make sure the hot surfaces are out of reach. Make sure the cords are out of reach also so that children can't pull the appliance down.
- If you are not using the heating appliance, unplug it.
- Adjust your hot water heater so that the water is 120 degrees Fahrenheit or cooler and can't scald a child who turns it on.
- Keep chemicals like bleach and drain cleaner out of children's reach.
- If you are holding a child or infant, put him down before you cook or work with something very hot.

FYI: Sunburns

Sunburns are a common type of burn, especially in children. They are typically mild but can be painful and cause blisters. The best treatment is prevention. You can prevent sunburn by following these suggestions:

- Keep infants younger than 6 months of age out of direct sunlight.
- For children older than 6 months of age, use sunscreen made for children.
- Put sunscreen on children 30 minutes before they go outside.

- Choose a water-resistant or waterproof sunscreen that blocks both UVA and UVB rays and has an SPF of at least 15.
- Reapply waterproof sunscreen every 2 hours, especially if children are playing in the water.
- Try to stay out of the sun between 10 AM and 4 PM.

Step 2: Be Safe

- Make sure the scene is safe.
- Get the first aid kit.
- Wear PPE.

Step 3: Phone 911

Phone 911

- If there is a fire
- If the child has a large burn
- If you are not sure what to do

Step 4: Act

Small Burns

Follow these steps for small burns:

Step	Action
1	Check the child and find all the burn areas.
2	If the burn area is small, cool it immediately with cold, but not ice-cold, water. Run cold water on the burn until it doesn't hurt.
3	You may cover the burn with a dry, nonstick sterile or clean dressing.

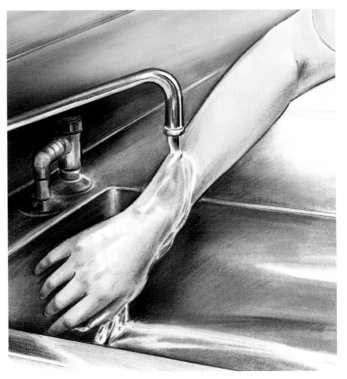

Figure 22. If the burn area is small, cool it immediately with cold, but not ice-cold, water.

Large Burns

Follow these steps for large burns:

Step	Action
1	If the child is on fire, put the fire out.
2	Check the child and find all the burn areas.
3	Remove jewelry and clothing that is not stuck to the skin.
4	Cover the child with a dry blanket.
5	Check for signs of shock.

Important

- If a child is on fire
  - Have the child stop, drop, and roll
  - Then cover the child with a wet blanket if available to put the fire out
  - Once the fire is out, remove the wet blanket
- Many people have heard about different ointments for burns. The only thing you should put on a burn is cold water and clean dressings unless you are given other instructions by a healthcare provider.

FYI

Cover the child with a dry blanket to keep the child warm, because once the skin has burned, the child can no longer control body temperature as well and often gets cold.

Electrical Injuries

Definitions and Key Facts

- Electricity can burn the body on the inside and outside. Electricity can stop breathing or cause an abnormal, deadly heart rhythm.
- Use cool water on burns. Ice can damage burned areas. If someone with a burn gets too cold, she can get hypothermia (low body temperature).

Step 1: Prevent

Use the Child and Infant Safety Checklist.

Step 2: Be Safe

- Make sure the scene is safe.
- Get the first aid kit and AED.
- Wear PPE.
- Stay clear of the injured child as long as he's in contact with a power source that is on. Electricity can travel from the source through the injured child to you. Turn off the main power switch only if you know how and can safely do so. Once the power is off, you may touch the injured child.

High voltage: If the electrical injury is caused by high voltage, such as a fallen power line, electricity can travel through everything that touches the power line or source (even a wooden stick). Wait until the power has been turned off to enter the area and provide help.

Step 3: Phone 911

Phone 911

- If a child has an electrical injury

Step 4: Act

Follow these steps to help a child with an electrical injury:

Step	Action
1	Look for burns and other injuries. • Electricity may leave only small marks on the body. • No one can tell how much damage there is inside the body based on the marks on the outside.
2	When it is safe to touch the injured child, see if he needs CPR. If he does, give CPR.

Eye Injuries

Definitions and Key Facts

Eye injuries may happen

- With a direct hit or punch to the eye or the side of the head
- When a ball or other object directly hits the eye
- When a high-speed object, such as a BB gun pellet, hits the eye
- When a stick or other sharp object punctures the eye
- When a small object, such as a piece of dirt, gets in the eye

Step 1: Prevent

Use the Child and Infant Safety Checklist to help keep a child safe.

Step 2: Be Safe

- Make sure the scene is safe.
- Get the first aid kit.
- Wear PPE.

Step 3: Phone 911

Phone 911

- If the eye is hit hard or punctured.
- If the irritant does not come out or if the child is in extreme pain, phone or ask someone to phone 911. Tell the child to keep her eyes closed.

Step 4: Act   Follow these steps to help a child with an eye injury:

Step	Action
1	Signs of an eye injury include • Pain • Trouble seeing • Bruising • Bleeding • Redness, swelling
2	If there is an irritant, such as sand, in the eye, use water to rinse the eye.
3	If the irritant does not come out or if the child is in extreme pain, phone or ask someone to phone 911. Tell the child to keep her eyes closed.

Fainting

Definitions and Key Facts

- Fainting is a short period when a child stops responding for less than a minute and then seems fine.
- This is usually caused by not enough blood going to the brain.
- Seconds before fainting, the child may feel dizzy.
- Fainting often occurs when the child
  - Stands without moving for a long time, especially if the weather is hot
  - Has a heart condition

Step 1: Prevent

If a child feels dizzy or weak, move her to someplace safe. If it's hot outside, giving the child something cool to drink may help.

Step 2: Be Safe

- Make sure the scene is safe.
- Get the first aid kit.

Step 3: Phone 911

Phone 911

- If the child faints and then starts to respond
- If the child stops responding

Step 4: Act   Follow these steps to help a child who faints:

Step	Action
1	If the child is dizzy and still responds, have her lie flat on the floor.
2	If a child faints and then starts to respond, ask the child to continue to lie flat on the floor until she can sit up and feels normal.
3	If the child fell, look for injuries caused by the fall.

Fever

Definitions and Key Facts

- Fever is a high body temperature. It's the body's natural way of fighting illness.
- Fever can be caused by an illness or infection.
- Some fevers are low and don't need first aid.
- Some children with a fever may have a seizure.
- You can take the child's temperature in several places. These places are recommended:
  - In the armpit
  - Under the tongue
  - In the ear
  - Across the forehead
- Glass can break and hurt the child. Use a non-glass thermometer.

Step 1: Prevent   You can't prevent fevers. Washing hands can help prevent illnesses from spreading.

Step 2: Be Safe   Keep a child with fever away from other children.

Step 3: Phone 911   Phone 911 if the child

- Has a seizure
- Has trouble breathing
- Shows signs of shock or dehydration
- Is hard to wake up

Step 4: Act

Follow these steps to help a child with a fever:

Step	Action
1	If the child feels hot or if you suspect a child has a fever, check the child's temperature.
2	Call the parent/guardian or healthcare provider if a child has a fever.
3	Give medicine to reduce fever only if the child's parent/guardian or healthcare provider tells you to do so and only if the medicine has been approved by the parent/guardian or healthcare provider.
4	Move the sick child away from any other children to help prevent other children becoming ill.

Important

Giving aspirin to children can be very dangerous and may lead to Reye's Syndrome. Only give aspirin if a healthcare provider specifically tells you to. Aspirin is different from ibuprofen or acetaminophen.

Frostbite

Definitions and Key Facts

- Cold-related emergencies may involve only part of the body or the whole body.
- A cold injury to part of the body is called frostbite. Cold injury to the whole body is called low body temperature, or hypothermia.
- Frostbite affects parts of the body that are exposed to the cold, such as the fingers, toes, nose, and ears.
- Frostbite typically occurs outside in cold weather. But it can also occur inside when people without gloves handle extremely cold materials.

Step 1: Prevent

- Make sure children wear appropriate clothing in cold weather.
- Watch small children closely if they are in very cold weather to make sure they stay warm.

Step 2: Be Safe

Make sure the scene is safe.

Step 3: Phone 911

Phone 911

- If you suspect frostbite

Step 4: Act   Follow these steps to help a child with frostbite:

Step	Action
1	Signs of frostbite include • Waxy, white, or grayish-yellow skin • Cold and numb body parts • Hard skin that doesn't move when you push it
2	Move the child to a warm place.
3	Remove tight clothing, rings, or bracelets from the frostbitten part.
4	Remove any wet clothing.
5	Do not try to thaw the frozen part if you think there may be a chance of the body part refreezing before you can get to medical care.

Head, Neck, and Spine Injuries

Definitions and Key Facts

- The bones of the spine protect the spinal cord. The spinal cord carries messages between the brain and the body.
- If the spine is damaged, the spinal cord may be injured. The child may not be able to move her legs or arms and may lose feeling in parts of the body. Some people call this a "broken back."
- Head injuries may occur if a child
  - Fell from a height
  - Was hit in the head
  - Was injured while diving
  - Suffered an electrical injury
  - Was involved in a car crash
  - Was riding a bicycle or motorbike involved in a crash, and has no helmet or a broken helmet

Step 1: Prevent   Use the Child and Infant Safety Checklist to help keep a child safe.

Step 2: Be Safe
- Make sure the scene is safe.
- Get the first aid kit.
- Wear PPE.

Step 3: Phone 911   Phone 911

- If you suspect a head, neck, or spine injury

Step 4: Act

Follow these steps to help a child with a head, neck, or spine injury:

Step	Action
1	Check an injured child to see if he • Does not respond or only moans or moves • Acts sleepy or confused • Vomits • Complains of a headache • Has trouble seeing • Has trouble walking or moving any part of the body • Has a seizure
2	Check an injured child to see if he • Has tingling or weakness in the extremities • Has pain or tenderness in the neck or back • Appears to be not fully alert • Has other painful injuries, especially of the head and neck
3	If you suspect any of these injuries, minimize movement of the head and neck.

Important

- You may cause further injury to the spinal cord if you bend, twist, or turn the child's head or neck. When you give first aid to someone with a possible spine injury, you must not bend, twist, or turn the head or neck unless it's necessary to provide CPR or if you need to move the child out of danger.
- If the child is vomiting or has fluids in her mouth, wear PPE and roll her onto her side.

Penetrating and Puncturing Injuries

Definitions and Key Facts

- An object such as a knife or sharp stick can cause a penetrating injury or an injury that punctures the skin.
- Leave it in place until a healthcare provider can treat the injury.

Step 1: Prevent

Use the Child and Infant Safety Checklist to create a safer environment.

Step 2: Be Safe

- Make sure the scene is safe.
- Get the first aid kit.
- Wear PPE.

Step 3: Phone 911

Phone 911

- If an object penetrates or punctures and gets stuck in a child

Step 4: Act

Follow these steps to help a child with a penetrating or puncturing injury:

Step	Action
1	Find the place on the child's body where the object has gone in.
2	Leave the object in the body.
3	Stop any bleeding you can see.
4	Have the child keep still until someone with more advanced training takes over.

Poison

Definitions and Key Facts

- This section will not deal with specific poisons. Instead it will cover general principles of first aid for a child exposed to a poison.
- A poison is anything a child swallows, breathes, or gets in the eyes or on the skin that causes sickness or death. Many products can poison children.
- The number for the American Association of Poison Control Centers is 1-800-222-1222.

Step 1: Prevent

To prevent poisonings, keep potentially dangerous items out of children's reach. Some examples include

- All medicine, including vitamins and supplements
- Mouthwash
- Lamp oil
- Cleaning supplies
- Chemicals

Use the Child and Infant Safety Checklist to create a safer environment.

Step 2: Be Safe

Make sure the scene is safe before you approach the child. Look out for spilled or leaking bottles or boxes.

- If there is a chemical spill or the child is in an unsafe area, try to move the child to an area with fresh air if you can do so safely.
- Ask everyone to move away from the area.
- Get the first aid kit.
- Wear PPE. Whenever possible, use a mask when giving breaths. This is especially important if the poison is on the child's lips or mouth and you need to give CPR.

Step 3: Phone 911

Phone 911 and check if the child needs CPR.

The 911 dispatcher can get help on the way quickly and often can also connect you to poison control.

When you phone 911, try to have the following information ready:

- What is the name of the poison? Can you describe it if you cannot name it?
- How much poison did the child touch, breathe, or swallow?
- About how old is the child? About how much does the child weigh?
- When did the poisoning happen?
- How is the child feeling or acting now?

Step 4: Act

Follow these steps to help a child who has a poison emergency:

Step	Action
1	Suspect that a child has been poisoned if • You see empty containers that used to have dangerous contents, such as pill, vitamin, or perfume bottles • A child has a chemical smell on his breath or body • You suspect the child has eaten parts of a plant • You smell something you suspect is poisonous or dangerous in the room with a child
2	Help the child take off contaminated clothing and jewelry if you can do so safely.
3	Run clean water over the skin, eyes, and other contaminated areas of the child's body for at least 20 minutes or until someone with more advanced training arrives and takes over.
4	Ask the child to blink as much as possible while rinsing his eyes.

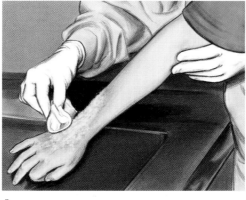
A

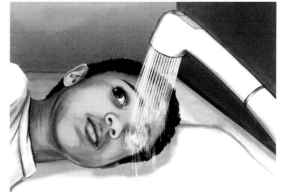
B

Figure 23. Remove poisons. **A,** Brush off any dry powder or solid substances. **B,** Rinse the eye.

Important	Some dispatchers may connect you to a poison control center. Only give medicines that the poison control center or dispatcher tells you to. The first aid instructions on the poison itself can be helpful but may be incomplete.

Seizure

Definitions and Key Facts	■ A seizure is abnormal electrical activity in the brain. Most seizures stop within a few minutes. A medical condition called epilepsy often causes seizures.
	
	■ Not all seizures are due to epilepsy. Some seizures happen when the heart suddenly stops beating. Seizures can also be caused by
	  – Head injury
	  – Low blood sugar
	  – Heat-related injury
	  – Poisons
	  – Very high fevers (in infants and young children)
	
	The child may bite his tongue during a seizure. You can give first aid for that injury after the seizure stops. After a seizure it is not unusual for the child to be confused or sleepy.

Step 1: Prevent	■ A child's first aid action plan for seizures may list possible triggers to avoid.
	
	■ Sometimes you can't prevent a seizure but you can prepare for one. Some children wet or soil their pants during a seizure.
	  – Protect a child's privacy and prevent discomfort by covering her pants with a blanket.
	  – Have a clean pair of pants for her to change into.

Step 2: Be Safe	■ Make sure the scene is safe. ■ Get the first aid kit. ■ Wear PPE.

Step 3: Phone 911	Phone 911
	
	  ■ If this is the child's first seizure
	  ■ If you are unsure whether the child has had a seizure before
	  ■ If your first aid action plan for this child says to phone 911
	  ■ If there is more than 1 seizure in a row or they do not stop

Step 4: Act   Follow these steps to help a child who is having a seizure:

Step	Action
1	Look for the following: • Loss of muscle control • Falling to the ground • Jerking arms, legs, or other body parts • Lost control of bowels or bladder • Biting the tongue (give any first aid for that after giving first aid for the seizure) • Stops responding
2	Protect the child by • Moving furniture or other objects out of the way • Placing a small towel or pad under the child's head if it's easy to do so • Removing any loose blankets around an infant or child
3	After the seizure • See if the child needs CPR • If the child is vomiting or has fluids in his mouth and you think that he does not have a head, neck, or spine injury, roll him onto his side

Important   There are many myths about what to do when a child has a seizure. Some tell you to do things that actually may hurt the child (such as putting something in her mouth). The action tables provide the correct information about caring for someone having a seizure.

Splinters

Definitions and Key Facts   Splinters are small pieces of wood or metal that stick under the skin.

Step 1: Prevent   Use the Child and Infant Safety Checklist to help keep a child safe.

Step 2: Be Safe
- Make sure the scene is safe.
- Get the first aid kit.
- Wear PPE.

Step 3: Phone 911   Usually, you will not need to phone 911 for a splinter.

Step 4: Act

Follow these steps to help a child with a splinter:

Step	Action
1	Find the splinter.
2	If the splinter is small, put sticky tape over the splinter and pull the tape off.
3	If tape doesn't pull it out, hold the end of the splinter with clean tweezers and gently pull it out.
4	After you have removed the splinter, clean the child's wound with water and soap if available.
5	If you can't get it out, leave it in, and clean the area with soap and water. Get medical care if the splinter • Is large • Is deeply embedded in the skin • Is difficult to remove • Is in the eye • Broke off, possibly leaving part of it in the wound • Becomes infected

FYI

- If the splinter is in the eye, see the section on eye injuries and follow those actions rather than these.
- Keep the splinter dry, because if it's wet, it will be harder to remove in one piece.
- Use tweezers only to pull it out gently, without digging.

Tooth Injuries

Definitions and Key Facts

- Children with a mouth injury may have broken, loose, or knocked-out teeth. This can be a choking hazard, especially for young children.
- When baby teeth come out, a little bit of blood is normal.

Step 1: Prevent

Use the Child and Infant Safety Checklist.

Step 2: Be Safe

- Make sure the scene is safe.
- Get the first aid kit.
- Wear PPE.

Step 3: Phone 911 Phone 911

▪ If there is severe bleeding

Step 4: Act Follow these steps for injuries to permanent teeth:

Step	Action
1	Check the child's mouth for any missing teeth, loose teeth, or parts of teeth.
2	If a tooth is loose, have the child bite down on a piece of gauze to keep the tooth in place and call the child's parent/guardian or dentist. Tell the child's parent/guardian to talk with a dentist if a child's tooth changes color after an injury. The change in color may happen quickly or may take up to a year.
3	If a tooth is chipped, gently wash the injured area with saline or clean water and call the child's parent/guardian or dentist.
4	If the child has lost a tooth, apply pressure to stop any bleeding at the tooth socket. Rinse the tooth in water, put the tooth in a cup of milk, and immediately take the child and tooth to a dentist or emergency department.

Important

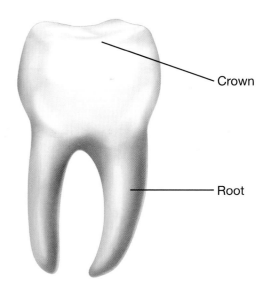

Crown

Root

Figure 24. Hold the tooth by the crown, not the root (the part that was in the gums). If it was a permanent tooth, there may be ligaments on the tooth that will help reattach it.

Keep the tooth out of the mouth.

FYI If a baby tooth is knocked out by accident, stop any bleeding with pressure and phone the dentist. You don't need to put the tooth in milk.

First Aid Review Questions

First Aid Steps

1. About what percentage of fatal injuries can be prevented by simple actions in the home, car, child care center, school, and playground?

    a. None

    b. At least half

    c. All

    d. One

2. Which of the following reduces the risk of SIDS?

    a. Putting the infant to sleep on her back

    b. Putting the infant to sleep on her stomach

    c. Making first aid action plans

    d. Ensuring that car seats are installed correctly

3. What is the most important step in preventing illness?

    a. Posting the poison control number near a phone

    b. Wearing a mask

    c. Putting all blood-containing material into a leak-proof bag

    d. Hand washing

4. The purpose of taking your gloves off properly is to keep blood or fluids on the gloves from touching your skin.

    a. True

    b. False

5. Why is it important to answer all of the dispatcher's questions?

    a. Because the 911 dispatcher needs to complete a survey

    b. Because it will get help to you as fast as possible

    c. To keep yourself safe so that you don't become a victim too

    d. So the dispatcher can give a report to the media

6. A person who reports possible child abuse is responsible for determining if the circumstances meet the legal definition of abuse.

    a. True

    b. False

7. Which of the following may be true about how a child acts when something is wrong?

    a. The child may act sick or hurt.

    b. The child may act younger than she is.

    c. The child may need for you to talk to her based on her behavior, not her age.

    d. All of the above

8. If you are not sure what is wrong with a child, you'll need to find the problem. What is the first step you should take?

   a. Checking for injuries or medical jewelry
   b. Checking for breathing
   c. Making sure the scene is safe
   d. Checking for a response (tap and shout)

| Group A1 |

1. What can stop most severe bleeding?

   a. Putting on gloves
   b. Putting direct pressure on the wound
   c. Applying an antibiotic cream
   d. Having the child lie down

2. Which of the following can be used as a dressing?

   a. A clean cloth
   b. A cold pack
   c. A dirty cloth
   d. A piece of tape

3. What should a child with a nosebleed do?

   a. Lie flat on the ground, facedown
   b. Lean backward as you apply pressure on the forehead
   c. Not be seen by a healthcare provider unless the bleeding lasts at least 4 hours
   d. Lean forward as you apply pressure on the soft part of the nose

4. One of the most common types of shock happens when a child has lost too much blood or water.

   a. True
   b. False

5. Which of the following is true of an epinephrine pen injection?

   a. It can be given through clothes or on bare skin.
   b. It should be used for every child with a rash.
   c. It can only be given through bare skin.
   d. It is always given in the side of the arm.

6. When a child has an asthma attack, what should you do?

   a. Give him something with sugar to drink.
   b. Leave him alone until his breathing gets better.
   c. Help the child use his prescription medication.
   d. Give him thrusts above the belly button.

7. If a child with low blood sugar is able to sit up and swallow, give her something containing sugar to eat or drink.

   a. True
   b. False

Group A2

1. Which of the following is true of heat stroke?

   a. Heat stroke can quickly turn into heat exhaustion.

   b. Heat stroke is never life threatening.

   c. Heat stroke is caused by vigorous exercise in a warm or hot environment.

   d. Heat stroke should be treated with warm water.

2. How can a child get hypothermia (low body temperature)?

   a. From walking in rain and wind without a jacket

   b. On a hot, sunny day

   c. When she doesn't have enough sugar in her blood

   d. After a seizure

3. In which of the following can a young child drown?

   a. A 5-gallon bucket

   b. A toilet

   c. A bathtub

   d. All of the above

Group B1

1. What should you do if a child has an injury that needs to be splinted?

   a. Place a plastic bag filled with warm water on the area to reduce swelling.

   b. Apply a splint only after an x-ray confirms that the bone is broken.

   c. Ideally, place the splint so that it supports the joints above and below the injury.

   d. Straighten the injured body part before using a splint.

2. What should you do when a child gets a small burn?

   a. Cool the area with cold, but not ice-cold, water.

   b. Cover the area with lots of cold cream and butter.

   c. Put the child in a bathtub filled with ice.

   d. Run warm water on the burn until it doesn't hurt.

Group B2

1. Which of the following is true of electrical injuries?

   a. Electrical injuries have no effect on the heart.

   b. Electrical injuries never cause injury inside the body.

   c. High-voltage electricity can travel through everything that touches the power line or source.

   d. All electrical injuries should be treated with ice.

2. What should you do if you suspect that a child has a fever?

   a. Allow the child to play with other children.

   b. Check his temperature.

   c. Put ice packs on him.

   d. Cover him with a blanket.

3. What is the most important thing to do for a child with a suspected head, neck, or spine injury?

   a. Have him sit up.

   b. Help him walk around.

   c. Minimize movement of the head or neck.

   d. Give him a sports drink.

Group B3

1. If a child has a penetrating injury, you should leave it in place until a healthcare provider can treat the injury.

   a. True

   b. False

2. What should you do if a child has a seizure?

   a. Protect the child by moving furniture or other objects out of the way.

   b. Put something big in his mouth so he won't bite his tongue.

   c. Pin down his arms and legs so he will not injure them or scare other children.

   d. Turn the child over so he is facedown.

3. What should you do if a child has a permanent tooth knocked out?

   a. Always hold the tooth by the root.

   b. Rinse the tooth with diet soda and place it in a cup of water.

   c. Immediately take the child and tooth to a dentist or emergency department.

   d. Attempt to put the tooth back in place.

Pediatric First Aid Skills Summary

Taking Off Gloves

- Grip one glove on the outside of the glove near the cuff and peel it down until it comes off inside out.
- Cup it with your other (gloved) hand.
- Place fingers of your bare hand inside the cuff of the glove that is still on your hand.
- Peel that glove off so that it comes off inside out, with the first glove inside it.
- If there is blood on the gloves, dispose of the gloves properly.

Finding the Problem

- Make sure the scene is safe and look for the cause of the problem. Wear PPE.
- Tap and shout. If the child doesn't respond, check to see if the child is breathing.
- If the child isn't breathing or is only gasping
  - Begin CPR
  - Send someone to phone 911 and get the AED
- If the child responds and is old enough to talk, ask what the problem is.
- If the child doesn't need CPR, look for signs of injury, such as bleeding.
- Look for medical information jewelry.

How to Stop Bleeding and Bandaging

- Make sure the scene is safe. Wear PPE.
- Place a dressing on the bleeding. Use the flat part of your fingers or the palm of your hand to apply pressure to the dressing.
- If the bleeding does not stop, add more dressings on top of the first and press harder.
- Keep pressure on the wound until it stops bleeding.
- If you can't keep pressure on the wound, wrap a bandage firmly over the dressings to hold them in place.

- Get the prescribed epinephrine pen.
- Take off the safety cap. Follow the instructions on the pen.
- Hold the epinephrine pen in your fist without touching either end because the needle comes out of one end.
- Push the end with the needle hard against the side of the child's thigh, about halfway between the hip and knee. Give the injection through clothes or on bare skin.
- Hold the pen in place for about 10 seconds.
- Remove the needle and pen by pulling straight out.

Child and Infant Safety Checklist

More than 9 million children between birth and age 19 are seen for injuries each year in US emergency departments. Injuries are the leading cause of death among children in this age group.

Safety checklists can help you learn risks for injury at home, in the car, at child care centers, at schools, and on playgrounds. Safety checklists also tell you what to do to reduce risk. But these only reduce risk. There is no such thing as a risk-free environment. That's why it's important to learn first aid.

Action	I follow this safety precaution (✔ = yes)	Purchase of safety item is required (✔ = yes)
Car Safety		
Birth to 12 months A child under 1 year of age should always ride in a rear-facing car seat. There are different types of rear-facing car seats: Infant-only seats can only be used rear-facing. Convertible and 3-in-1 car seats typically have higher height and weight limits for the rear-facing position, allowing you to keep your child rear-facing for a longer period of time.		
1 to 4 years Keep a child rear-facing as long as possible. It's the best way to keep him or her safe. The child should remain in a rear-facing car seat until he or she reaches the top height or weight limit allowed by the car seat's manufacturer. Once the child outgrows the rear-facing car seat, the child is ready to travel in a forward-facing car seat with a harness.		
4 to 6 years Keep a child in a forward-facing car seat with a harness until he or she reaches the top height or weight limit allowed by the car seat's manufacturer. Once the child outgrows the forward-facing car seat with a harness, it's time to travel in a booster seat, but still in the back seat.		

6 to 12 years Keep a child in a booster seat until he or she is big enough to fit in a seat belt properly. For a seat belt to fit properly, the lap belt must lie snugly across the upper thighs, not the stomach. The shoulder belt should lie snugly across the shoulder and chest and should not cross the neck or face. Remember: The child should still ride in the back seat because it's safer there.		
13 years and older A **seat belt** should lie across the upper thighs and be snugly across the shoulder and chest to restrain the child safely in a crash. It should not rest on the stomach area or across the neck.		
1. Never leave children alone in or around cars, even for a minute.		
2. Put something you'll need, like your cell phone, handbag, employee ID, or briefcase, on the floorboard in the back seat so that you always look in the back seat before locking up the car to prevent accidentally leaving a child in the car.		
3. Make sure all child passengers have left the vehicle after it is parked.		
4. Keep a large stuffed animal in the child's car seat when it's not occupied. When the child is placed in the seat, put the stuffed animal in the front passenger seat. It's a visual reminder that any time the stuffed animal is up front, the child is in the back seat in a child safety seat.		
5. Make arrangements with your child's child care center or babysitter that you will always call if your child will not be there on a particular day as scheduled.		
6. Keep vehicles locked at all times, even in the garage or driveway, and always set your parking brake.		
7. Keys and remote openers should never be left within reach of children.		
General Indoor Safety		
8. Place a sticker with emergency phone numbers near or on the phone. Include numbers for the EMS system, police, fire department, local hospital or physician, and poison control center, as well as your telephone number.		
9. Install smoke detectors in the hallway outside areas where children sleep or nap and on each floor at the head of stairs. Test the alarm monthly and replace batteries once a year (for example, in the fall when the time changes from daylight saving time).		
10. Install carbon monoxide detectors and test monthly.		
11. Make sure that there is an emergency exit, preferably 2, from the home, child care center, classroom, or other area where children are likely to be present. Make sure nothing is blocking the exit(s).		

12. Develop and practice a fire escape plan.		
13. Make sure that a working fire extinguisher is available, especially in areas of greatest risk of fire like the kitchen, furnace room, and near the fireplace.		
14. Make sure that all space heaters are safety approved. They should be in safe operating condition. They should be placed out of a child's reach and at least 3 feet from curtains, papers, and furniture. The heaters should have protective covers.		
15. Make sure all wood-burning stoves and fireplaces are inspected yearly and vented properly. Place stoves out of a child's reach.		
16. Make sure that electrical cords are not frayed or overloaded. Place out of a child's reach.		
17. Keep matches and lighters up high, out of children's sight and reach.		
18. Supervise children if a live candle is in the room. Blow out all candles when you leave the room or go to bed. Avoid the use of candles in the bedroom and other areas where people may fall asleep.		
19. Have flashlights and battery-powered lighting to use during a power outage.		
20. Install "shock stops" (plastic outlet plugs) or outlet covers on all electrical outlets.		
21. To prevent falls, always keep one hand on an infant sitting or lying on a high surface such as a changing table. Never leave an infant alone on a changing table, couch, bed, or other furniture.		
22. Always put an infant in a carrier on the floor.		
23. Keep halls and stairs lighted to prevent falls.		
24. Put toddler gates at the top and bottom of stairs. (Do not use accordion-type gates with wide spaces at the top. The child's head could become trapped in such a gate, and the child could strangle.)		
25. Infants and children should use stationary activity centers. Ideally, infant walkers will be avoided because they can lead to injuries.		
26. To prevent falls, put locks (available at hardware stores) on all windows. Put gates on the lower part of open windows.		
27. Tie up blind and window curtain cords.		
28. Store medicines and vitamins in child-resistant containers out of a child's reach. Lock drawers and cabinets.		

29. Store cleaning products out of a child's sight and reach.		
a. Store and label all household poisons in their original containers in high locked cabinets (not under sinks).		
b. Do not store chemicals or poisons in soda bottles.		
c. Store cleaning products away from food.		
30. Install safety latches or locks on cabinets that contain potentially dangerous items and are within a child's reach.		
31. Keep purses that contain vitamins, medicines, cigarettes, matches, jewelry, and calculators (which have easy-to-swallow button batteries) out of a child's reach.		
32. Install a lock or hook-and-eye latch on the door to the basement or garage to keep children from entering those areas. Put a lock at the top of the doorframe.		
33. Keep plants that may be harmful out of a child's reach. (Many plants are poisonous. Check with your poison control center.)		
34. Make sure that toy chests have lightweight lids, no lids, or safe-closing hinges.		
35. Follow age recommendations on toy labels.		
36. Keep all small items (including food items) that can choke a child out of reach. Test toys for size with a toilet paper roll. If the toy can fit inside the roll, it can choke a child.		
SIDS Prevention		
37. Place healthy full-term infants on their backs on a firm mattress to sleep.		
38. Make sure the crib is safe:		
a. The crib mattress should fit snugly, with no more than 2 fingers' width between the mattress and crib railing.		
b. The distance between crib slats should be less than 2⅜ inches (so the infant's head won't be caught).		
c. Keep all loose blankets, toys, etc out of the bed.		
d. Keep hanging crib toys out of reach.		
39. Infants need their own infant beds. The American Academy of Pediatrics does not recommend any specific bed sharing arrangements as safe.		
40. Use a crib in good repair. Avoid portable bed rails.		
41. Check to see if the crib or mattress has been recalled.		

Kitchen Safety		
42. To reduce the risk of burns		
a. Keep hot liquids, foods, and cooking utensils out of a child's reach.		
b. Put hot liquids and food away from the edge of the table.		
c. Cool on back burners when possible, and turn pot handles toward the center of the stove.		
d. Avoid using tablecloths and placemats that can be pulled, spilling hot liquids or food.		
e. Keep high chairs and stools away from the stove.		
f. Do not keep snacks near the stove.		
g. Do not hold infants or children while cooking or carrying hot foods or liquids.		
43. Keep knives and other sharp objects out of a child's reach.		
Bathroom Safety		
44. Bathe children in no more than 1 or 2 inches of water. Stay with infants and young children throughout bath time. Do not leave small infants or toddlers in the bathtub in the care of young siblings.		
45. Use skidproof mats or stickers in the bathtub and put a cushioned cover over faucets.		
46. Adjust the maximum temperature of the water heater to 120 degrees Fahrenheit (48.9 degrees Celsius) or below. Test temperature with a thermometer.		
47. Keep electrical appliances (such as radios, hair dryers, and space heaters) out of the bathroom or unplugged, away from water, and out of a child's reach.		
Firearms		
48. If firearms are stored in the home, keep them locked and out of a child's sight and reach. Lock and unload guns individually before storing them. Store ammunitions separate from the firearms.		
Outdoor Safety		
49. Make sure playground equipment is assembled and anchored correctly according to the manufacturer's instructions. The playground should have a level, cushioned surface, such as sand or wood chips.		

50. Make sure your child knows the rules of safe bicycling:
 	
    a. Wear a protective helmet.
 	
    b. Use the correct-size bicycle.
 	
    c. Ride on the right side of the road (with traffic).
 	
    d. Use hand signals and wear bright or reflective clothing.
 	
    e. Never bicycle in the dark or fog.
 	
    f. Young children riding alone should only bike on sidewalks or paths.		

51. Do not allow children to play with fireworks.		

52. Make sure your child is properly protected while roller skating or skateboarding:
 	
    a. Wear a helmet and protective pads on the knees and elbows.
 	
    b. Skate only in rinks or parks that are free of traffic.		

53. Make sure your child is properly protected while participating in contact sports:
 	
    a. Proper adult instruction and supervision are provided.
 	
    b. Appropriate safety equipment is used.		

54. To reduce the risk of animal bites, teach your child
 	
    a. How to handle and care for a pet
 	
    b. To avoid unfamiliar animals
 	
    c. To approach dogs calmly and slowly, and check with the owner first before approaching or petting		

55. If you have a home swimming pool, make sure the pool is totally enclosed with fencing that is at least 5 feet high and that all gates are self-closing and self-latching. There should be no direct access (without a locked gate) from the home into the pool area. In addition:
 	
    a. An adult must always supervise children while they swim. Never allow a child to swim alone.
 	
    b. All adults and older children should learn CPR.
 	
    c. Pools and nearby properties should be protected from use by unsupervised children.
 	
    d. Empty and turn over wading pools as soon as children are done using them.		

56. Protect children from sunburns:
 	
    a. Keep infants less than 6 months of age out of direct sunlight.
 	
    b. For children older than 6 months of age, use sunscreen made for children.
 	
    c. Put sunscreen on children 30 minutes before they go outside.
 	
    d. Choose a water-resistant or waterproof sunscreen that blocks both UVA and UVB rays and has an SPF of at least 15.
 	
    e. Reapply waterproof sunscreen every 2 hours, especially if children are playing in the water.
 	
    f. Try to stay out of the sun between 10 AM and 4 PM.		

The following sources were used in compiling the checklist:

1. National Highway Traffic Safety Administration

2. Centers for Disease Control and Prevention

3. American Academy of Pediatrics

4. Safe Kids USA

5. KidsAndCars.Org

6. National Rifle Association

7. National Fire Protection Association

The following sources were used in compiling the abuse information:

1. About Shaken Baby

2. National Center on Shaken Baby Syndrome

3. The Maryland and Oregon state governments

4. The National Institutes of Health

5. The Mayo Clinic

How Children Act and Tips for Interacting With Them

Children who are ill, injured, or afraid often do not act their age. Instead, they may act like a younger child. Respond to ill, injured, or frightened children based on their behavior, not their age.

The following table explains the characteristics and interaction tips for children of different ages:

Category	Age	Characteristics	Interaction Tips

Infants	Birth to 1 year	• Infants less than 4 months of age may not be able to hold head up
		• Cannot talk
		• Cry to tell you they are
		  – Hungry
		  – Tired
		  – Wet
		  – Want to be held
		  – Scared
		  – Hurt
			• Support the head when you lift or carry an infant less than 4 months of age.
			• Use a soft, quiet voice when you talk to an infant.
			• Use gentle motions when you approach an infant.
			• Keep the infant warm but not overly hot.

Toddlers	1 to 3 years	• Learning to talk
		• Active, moving around and making noise
		• May bite other children when frustrated
		• A toddler who is not active or is acting differently than usual may be
		  – Sick
		  – Hurt
		  – Afraid
		  – Tired
			• Toddlers may not speak well themselves.
			• They can often understand what others say.
			• They may be afraid of adults they do not know.
			• You may need to give extra comfort when a healthcare provider arrives to care for a toddler.

(continued)

(continued)

Category	Age	Characteristics	Interaction Tips
Young children	4 to 10 years	• Developmental stages overlap greatly within this age group • Often pick up on the feelings of adults around them • Can understand simple explanations • Fear separation from caregivers and friends	• Stay calm. • Use simple words to tell young children what is happening.

Adolescents	11 to 18 years	• Understand almost everything around them
		• Often act without worrying about consequences of their actions
		• May take risks such as experimenting with drugs, alcohol, and driving cars
		• May worry about
		  – How others view them
		  – Whether an injury will be permanent
		  – Getting into trouble because of an injury
		• May not share information with a first aid rescuer and especially the adolescent's own parent or guardian
			• Tell them what you are doing to help them.
			• Reassure them without talking down to them.

Children with special needs	Any age	• Have physical, mental, or emotional needs that require special care	• Work with family members or other caregivers to know how to use medical devices or medicines.

CPR, AED, and Choking

CPR stands for cardiopulmonary resuscitation. CPR consists of pushing on the chest and giving breaths. In this section, you'll learn both when to give CPR and how to do it.

- First, you'll learn how to actually give CPR.
- Then you'll learn about AEDs.
- Once you know how to give CPR and use an AED, you'll learn about when to give CPR.
- Finally, you'll learn how to put it all together—how to figure out if CPR is needed, and then give it.
- After you learn CPR for a child, you'll learn how to help a choking child.
- After you learn CPR for an infant, you'll learn how to help a choking infant.
- After you learn CPR for an adult, you'll learn how to help a choking adult.

Some key parts of learning how and when to give CPR are as follows:

Give CPR	This includes how to push on the chest and how to give breaths.
Use an AED	An AED can help shock a heart and help it work properly again. You may or may not have access to an AED, but if you do, use it.
Assess and Phone 911	You will learn when to give CPR and when you need to phone 911.
Put It All Together	This is when you put all your skills together. First you assess, or figure out, whether a person needs CPR, and then, if CPR is needed, you can give it.
CPR AED Testing	Once you have finished practicing, you'll be tested on both figuring out if a person needs CPR and how to give it.

What You Will Learn   You'll learn when and how to provide CPR and use AEDs. You'll also learn what to do when someone is choking.

Topics Covered

- CPR and AED for Children
- How to Help a Choking Child
- CPR for Infants
- How to Help a Choking Infant
- CPR and AED for Adults
- How to Help a Choking Adult

CPR and AED for Children

What You Will Learn

In this section you'll learn when CPR is needed, how to give CPR to a child, and how to use an AED.

Definitions and Key Facts

CPR stands for cardiopulmonary resuscitation. It consists of pushing on the chest (compressions) and giving breaths.

CPR is given to someone whose heart has stopped pumping blood.

For purposes of this course, a child is someone who is older than 1 year and has not yet reached puberty. If you are in doubt about whether someone is an adult or child, treat as an adult.

A child who "responds" moves, speaks, blinks, or otherwise reacts to you when you tap him and ask if he's OK. A child who doesn't "respond" does nothing when you tap him and ask if he's OK.

Topics Covered

- Give CPR: Compressions and Breaths
- Use an AED
- Assess and Phone 911
- Put It All Together

Give CPR: Compressions and Breaths

Compressions

Definitions and Key Facts

Pushing hard and fast on the chest (compressions) is the most important part of CPR. When you push on the chest, you pump blood to the brain and heart. People often don't push hard enough because they're afraid of hurting the child. An injury is unlikely, but it is better than death. It's better to push too hard than not hard enough.

Action: Push Hard and Push Fast

Follow these steps to push hard and push fast:

Step	Action
1	Make sure the child is lying on her back on a firm, flat surface.
2	Move clothes out of the way.
3	Put the heel of one hand on the lower half of the breastbone.
4	Push straight down **about 2 inches** at a rate of **at least 100 compressions a minute.**
5	After each compression, let the **chest come back up** to its normal position.

FYI

Use 1 hand for compressions. If you can't push down about 2 inches with 1 hand, use 2. One hand is not better than 2 or vice versa. Do what's necessary to push the chest down about 2 inches.

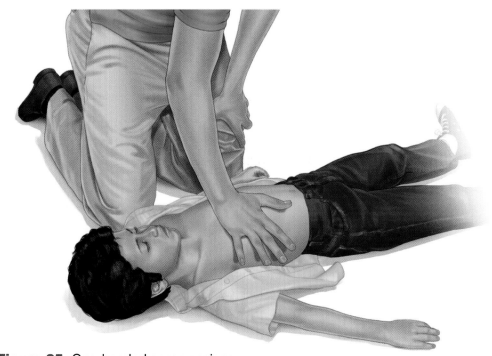

Figure 25. One-handed compressions.

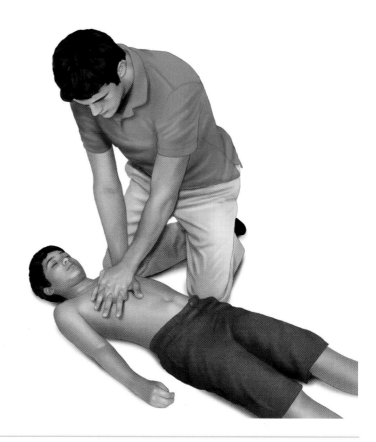

Figure 26. Two-handed compressions.

FYI

Compressions are important in CPR, and doing them right is tiring. The more tired you are, the less effective your compressions are. If someone else knows CPR, take turns. Switch about every 2 minutes, moving quickly so that the pause in compressions is as short as possible. Remind each other to push down **about 2 inches,** to push at a rate of **at least 100 compressions a minute,** and to let the **chest come back up** to its normal position after each compression.

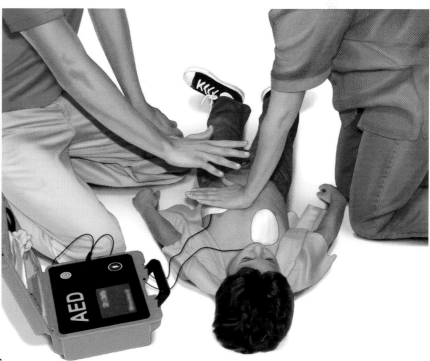

Figure 27.
Switch rescuers.

Definitions and Key Facts

Children often have healthy hearts. Usually, a child's heart stops because she can't breathe or is having trouble breathing. As a result, it's very important to give breaths as well as compressions to a child.

You may have heard of Hands-Only™ CPR, which is CPR without mouth-to-mouth breaths. However, Hands-Only CPR is recommended when you see an adult collapse. For children, we recommend traditional CPR, which includes giving breaths.

Your breaths need to make the child's chest rise. When the chest rises, you know the child has gotten enough air. Compressions are the most important part of CPR. If you are also able to give breaths, you will help the child even more.

Action: Open the Airway

Before giving breaths, open the airway. Follow these steps to open the airway:

Step	Action
1	Put one hand on the forehead and the fingers of your other hand on the bony part of the child's chin.
2	Tilt the head back and lift the chin.

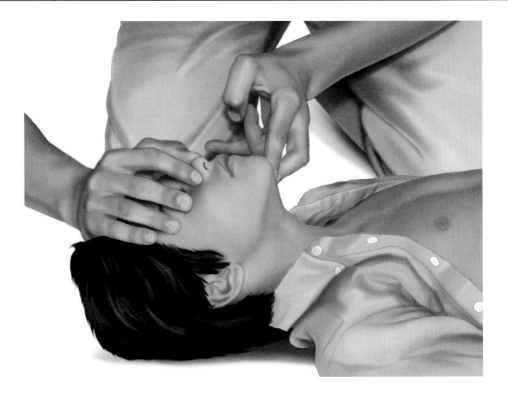

Figure 28. Open the airway by tilting the head and lifting the chin.

Important

Avoid pressing on the soft part of the neck or under the chin.

**Action:
Give Breaths**

Follow these steps to give breaths to a child:

Step	Action
1	While holding the airway open, pinch the nose closed.
2	Take a breath. Cover the child's mouth with your mouth.
3	**Give 2 breaths** (blow for 1 second each). Watch for **the chest to begin to rise** as you give each breath.

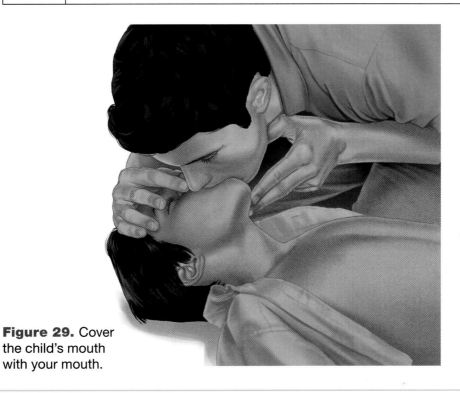

Figure 29. Cover the child's mouth with your mouth.

Important

If you give a child a breath and the chest doesn't rise, reopen the airway by allowing the head to go back to the normal position. Then open the airway again by tilting the head and lifting the chin. Then give another breath. Make sure the chest rises.

Don't interrupt compressions for more than 10 seconds to give breaths. If the chest doesn't rise within 10 seconds, begin pushing hard and pushing fast on the chest again.

Using a Mask

**Definitions and
Key Facts**

Giving breaths to another person is usually quite safe. During CPR there is very little chance that you will catch a disease. Even so, some child care centers require rescuers to have masks.

Masks are made of firm plastic; they fit over the child's mouth or mouth and nose. You may need to put the mask together before you use it.

Actions

Follow these steps to give breaths with a mask:

Step	Action
1	Put the mask over the child's mouth and nose.
2	Tilt the head and lift the chin while pressing the mask against the child's face. It is important to make an airtight seal between the child's face and the mask while you lift the chin to keep the airway open.
3	Give 2 breaths. Watch for the chest to begin to rise as you give each breath.

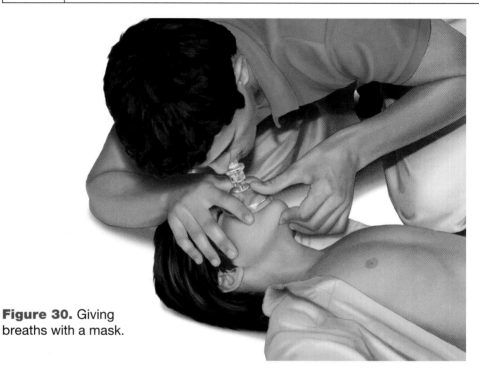

Figure 30. Giving breaths with a mask.

FYI

If the mask has a pointed end

- Put the narrow end of the mask at the top (bridge) of the nose
- Position the wide end to cover the mouth

Use an AED

Definitions and Key Facts

If you start CPR right away and use an automated external defibrillator (AED) within a few minutes, you will have the best chance of saving a life.

AEDs are safe, accurate, and easy to use. The most common ways to turn on an AED are to push an "ON" button or lift the lid of the AED. Once you turn on the AED, it will tell you everything you need to do.

The AED will figure out if the child needs a shock and will tell you to give one if needed. It will even tell you when to make sure that no one is touching the child. The pads used to shock the child have a diagram showing you where to place them. Follow the diagram.

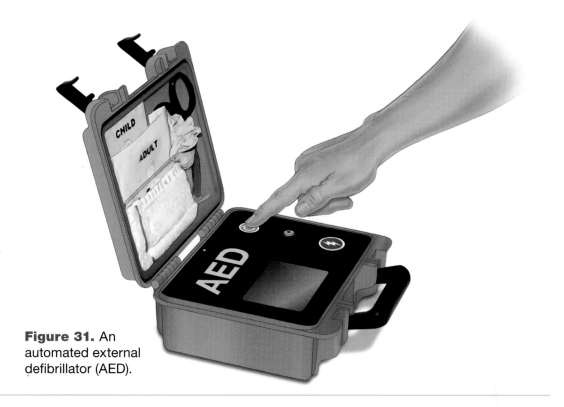

Figure 31. An automated external defibrillator (AED).

Action

Use an AED on any child who needs CPR. Follow these 4 simple steps for using an AED on a child:

Step	Action
1	Turn the AED on.
2	Look for child pads or for a child key or switch.
3	Use the child pads or turn the child key or switch.
4	Follow the prompts you see and hear.

Important

If there are no child pads or if there isn't a child key or switch, use the adult pads. Also, if the child is older than 8 years, use adult pads. (If you think the child might be 8 or older, assume he is, and use the adult pads.) When you put the pads on the chest, make sure they don't touch each other. If a child is very small, you may need to put one pad on the child's chest and the other on the child's back.

If you have access to an AED, use it as quickly as possible. Make sure no one is touching the child just before pushing the "SHOCK" button. If you can't find an AED quickly, don't wait. Start CPR.

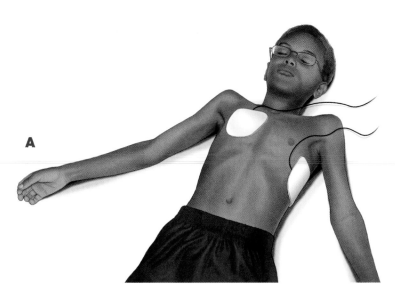

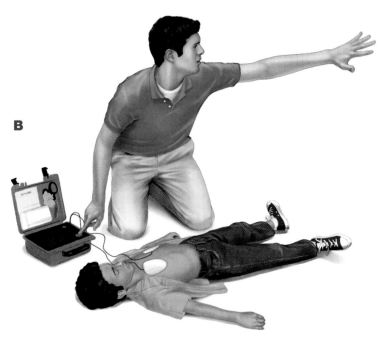

Figure 32. A, Placing child pads on a child. **B,** Making sure no one is touching the child.

Assess and Phone 911

Definitions and Key Facts

Now that you've learned how to give CPR, it's time to learn when to give CPR. If a child doesn't respond and if that child isn't breathing or is only gasping, then you need to give CPR.

If you are not sure whether to give CPR, go ahead and give it. It's better to give CPR to someone who doesn't need it than not to give it to someone who does need it.

Action: Make Sure the Scene Is Safe

Before you give CPR, make sure the scene is safe. Look for anything nearby that might hurt you. You don't want to hurt yourself.

Action: Tap and Shout

Check if the child responds. Tap him and shout, "Are you OK?" If he doesn't move, speak, blink, or otherwise react, then he is not responding.

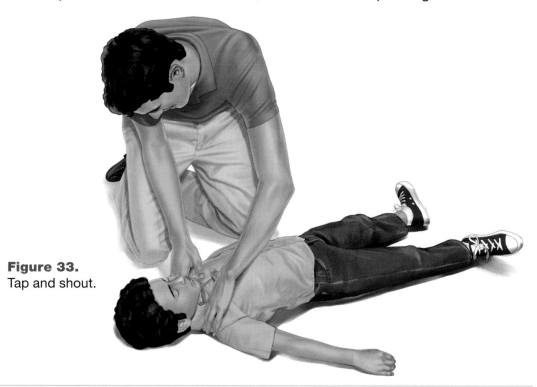

Figure 33.
Tap and shout.

Action: Yell for Help

Yell for help. If someone comes, have that person phone 911 and get an AED. Whether or not someone comes, check the child's breathing next.

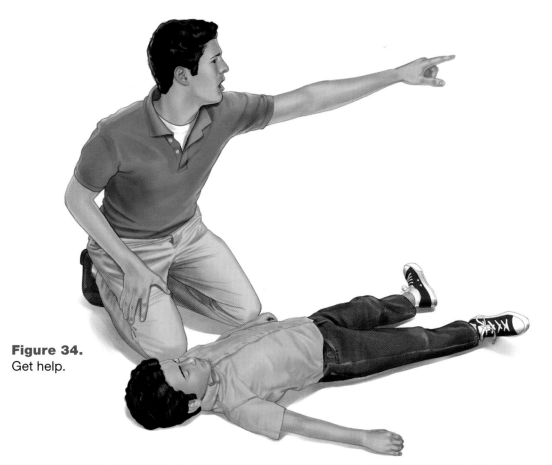

Figure 34.
Get help.

Action: Check Breathing	If the child doesn't respond, check his breathing. If the child isn't breathing at all or if he is only "gasping," then he needs CPR.

A person who gasps usually appears to be drawing air in very quickly. He may open his mouth and move the jaw, head, or neck. Gasps may appear forceful or weak, and some time may pass between gasps, as they usually happen at a slow rate. The gasp may sound like a snort, snore, or groan. Gasping is not regular or normal breathing. It is a sign of cardiac arrest in someone who doesn't respond.

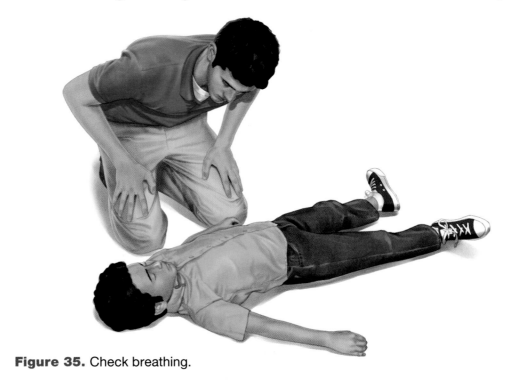

Figure 35. Check breathing.

Put It All Together (*Skill You Will Demonstrate)

Definitions and Key Facts	Since children's hearts are often healthy and since breathing trouble is often the cause of the child's heart problem, it's important to get air to the child as fast as possible. For this reason, you should give 5 sets of CPR before phoning for help or getting an AED. (If someone else is nearby, send that person to phone for help and to get an AED as quickly as possible.)
	Compressions are very important; they are the core of CPR. Try not to interrupt compressions for more than a few seconds, even when you give breaths.
Action: Give 5 Sets of CPR	When doing CPR, you **give sets of 30 compressions and 2 breaths.** Push down **about 2 inches** at a rate of **at least 100 times a minute.** After each push, let the **chest come back** up to its normal position.
	If the child doesn't respond and isn't breathing or is only gasping, give him 5 sets of CPR (1 set = 30 compressions and 2 breaths).

Action: Phone and Get an AED	After 5 sets of CPR, phone 911 and get an AED, if no one has done this yet. As soon as you have the AED, use it.
Action: Keep Going	After phoning 911, keep giving sets of 30 compressions and 2 breaths until the child begins to respond or until someone with more advanced training arrives and takes over.
FYI: Answering Dispatcher Questions	You need to stay on the phone until the 911 dispatcher (operator) tells you to hang up. The dispatcher will ask you about the emergency. She may also tell you how to help the child until someone with more advanced training arrives and takes over. Answering the dispatcher's questions will not delay the arrival of help. If you can, take the phone with you so that you are beside the child while you talk to the dispatcher.

Action: Child CPR

No response + **No breathing or only gasping** = **GIVE CPR**

Follow these steps for child CPR:

Step	Action
1	Make sure the scene is safe.
2	Tap and shout.
3	Yell for help.
4	Check breathing.
5	If the child isn't responding and either isn't breathing or is only gasping, **give 5 sets of 30 compressions and 2 breaths; then phone 911 and get an AED.**
6	Keep giving **sets of compressions and breaths** until the child starts to speak, breathe, or move, or until someone with more advanced training arrives and takes over.

Important

If another person is with you when you give CPR—or if you can yell for help and get someone to come help you—then send the other person to phone 911 while you start pushing hard and fast and giving breaths. **You give compressions and breaths; the other person phones and gets the AED.**

Child CPR AED Skills Summary

Step	Action
1	**Make sure the scene is safe.**
2	**Tap and shout.** ▪ Check to see if the person responds. ▪ If the person doesn't respond, go to Step 3.
3	**Yell for help.** ▪ See if someone can help you. ▪ Have that person phone 911 and get an AED.
4	**Check breathing.** ▪ Make sure the child is on a firm, flat surface. ▪ See if the child is not breathing at all or only gasping. No response + No breathing or only gasping = **GIVE CPR**
5	**Give CPR. Give 5 sets of 30 compressions and 2 breaths, and then phone 911 and get an AED (if no one has done this yet).** ▪ Compressions: – Move clothes out of the way. – Put the heel of one hand on the lower half of the breastbone. – Push straight down about 2 inches at a rate of at least 100 compressions a minute. – After each compression, let the chest come back up to its normal position. – Compress the chest 30 times. ▪ Breaths: – After 30 compressions, open the airway with a head tilt–chin lift. – After the airway is open, take a normal breath. – Pinch the nose shut. Cover the child's mouth with your mouth. – Give 2 breaths (blow for 1 second each). Watch for the chest to begin to rise as you give each breath. ▪ AED: – Use it as soon as you have it. – Turn it on by lifting the lid or pressing the "ON" button. – Use child pads or child key or switch. (Use adult pads if no child pads are available.) – Follow the prompts.
6	**Keep going.** ▪ Keep giving sets of compressions and breaths until the child starts to breathe or move, or until someone with more advanced training arrives and takes over.

How to Help a Choking Child

What You Will Learn In this section you'll learn the signs of choking and how to help a choking child.

Definitions and Key Facts Choking is when food or another object gets stuck in the airway or throat. The object stops air from getting to the lungs.

Some choking is mild and some is severe. If it's severe, act fast. Get the object out so the child can breathe.

Topics Covered
- Mild vs Severe Choking
- How to Help a Choking Child
- How to Help a Choking Child Who Stops Responding

Mild vs Severe Choking

Action Use the following table to figure out if a child has mild or severe choking and what you should do:

If the child	The block in the airway is	And you should
• Can make sounds • Can cough loudly	Mild	• Stand by and let her cough • If you are worried about her breathing, phone 911
• Cannot breathe or • Has a cough that has no sound or • Cannot talk or make a sound or • Makes the choking sign	Severe	• Act quickly • Follow the steps to help a choking child

A child who is choking might use the choking sign (holding the neck with one or both hands).

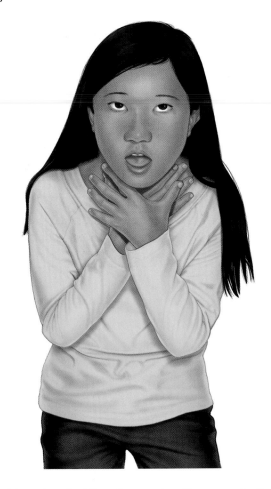

Figure 36. The choking sign: holding the neck with one or both hands.

How to Help a Choking Child

**Definitions and
Key Facts**

When a child has severe choking, give thrusts slightly above the belly button. These thrusts are sometimes called the Heimlich maneuver. Like a cough, each thrust pushes air from the lungs. This can help remove an object that is blocking the airway.

Action: Help a Choking Child

Follow these steps to help a choking child:

Step	Action
1	If you think the child is choking, ask, "Are you choking?" If she nods yes, tell her you are going to help.
2	**Get behind her.** Wrap your arms around her so that your hands are in front.
3	**Make a fist** with one hand.
4	Put the thumb side of your fist slightly above the belly button and well below the breastbone.
5	**Grasp the fist with your other hand** and give quick upward thrusts into the abdomen.
6	**Give thrusts** until the object is forced out and she can breathe, cough, or talk, or until she stops responding.

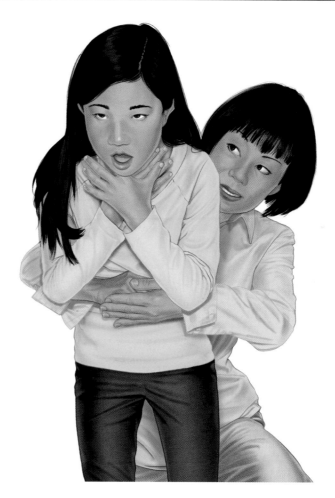

Figure 37. Helping a choking child.

Action: Adapt to a Child's Size

If the choking child is very large and you can't wrap your arms fully around the waist, give thrusts on the chest instead of thrusts on the abdomen.

If the child is small, you may have to kneel to get into the correct position.

Follow the same steps except for the location where you place your arms and hands. Put your arms under the child's armpits and your hands on the lower half of the breastbone. Pull straight back to give the chest thrusts.

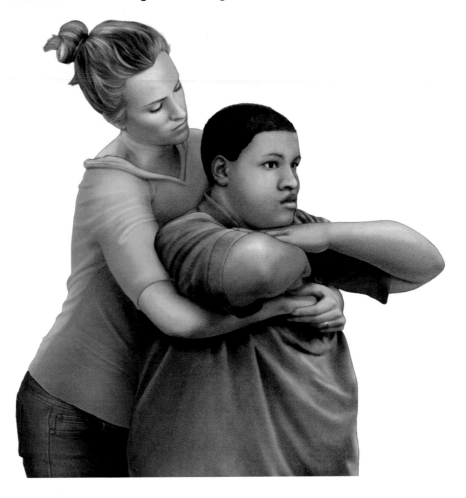

Figure 38. Chest thrusts on a choking large child.

FYI

A child who has been given thrusts should see a healthcare provider.

How to Help a Choking Child Who Stops Responding

Definitions and Key Facts

If you give a child thrusts but you can't remove the object blocking the airway, the child will stop responding. Pushing on his chest may force the object out.

Action: Help a Child Who Stops Responding

Follow these steps if the child stops responding:

Step	Action
1	Lower the child to a firm, flat surface.
2	Tap and shout.
3	**Yell for help.**
4	**Check breathing.**
5	**Give 30 compressions.**
6	After 30 compressions, open the airway. **If you see an object in the mouth, take it out.**
7	**Give 2 breaths.**
8	**Repeat** giving **sets of 30 compressions and 2 breaths**, checking the mouth for objects after each set of compressions.
9	**After 5 sets of 30 compressions and 2 breaths, phone** 911 and get an AED.
10	**Give sets of 30 compressions and 2 breaths,** checking the mouth for objects after each set of compressions until the child starts to respond or until someone with more advanced training arrives and takes over.

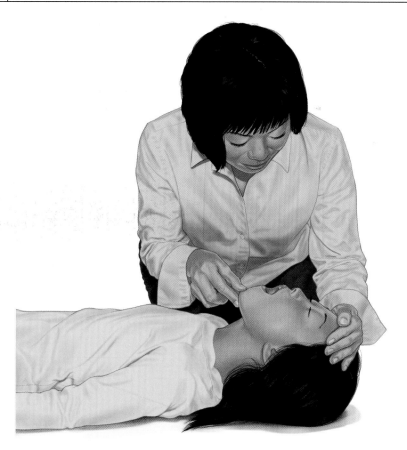

Figure 39. Open the child's mouth wide and look for the object.

Important

If another person is with you when the child stops responding—or if you can yell for help and get someone to come help you—send the other person to phone 911 and get an AED while you start pushing hard and fast and giving breaths. **You give compressions and breaths; the other person phones and gets the AED.**

CPR for Infants

What You Will Learn In this section you'll learn when to give CPR and how to give CPR to an infant.

Definitions and Key Facts CPR is the act of pushing hard and pushing fast on the chest and giving breaths. CPR is given to someone whose heart has stopped pumping blood.

For purposes of this course, an infant is someone who is younger than 1 year.

An infant who "responds" moves, makes sounds, blinks, or otherwise reacts to you when you tap him and shout his name. An infant who doesn't "respond" does nothing when you tap him and shout.

Topics Covered
- Give CPR: Compressions and Breaths
- Assess and Phone 911
- Put It All Together

Give CPR: Compressions and Breaths

Compressions

Definitions and Key Facts Pushing hard and fast on the chest (compressions) is the most important part of CPR. When you push on the chest, you pump blood to the brain and heart.

People often don't push hard enough because they're afraid of hurting the infant. An injury is unlikely, but it is better than death. It's better to push too hard than not hard enough.

If possible, place the infant on a firm, flat surface above the ground, such as a table. This makes it easier to give CPR.

Follow these steps to push hard and push fast:

Step	Action
1	Make sure the infant is lying on her back on a firm, flat surface. If possible, use a surface above the ground.
2	Move clothes out of the way.
3	Put 2 fingers of one hand on the breastbone just below the nipple line.
4	Press the infant's chest straight down about **1½ inches** at a rate of **at least 100 compressions a minute.**
5	After each compression, let the **chest come back up** to its normal position.

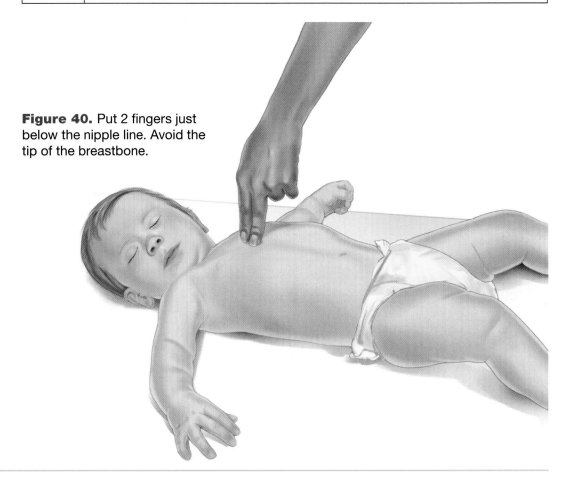

Figure 40. Put 2 fingers just below the nipple line. Avoid the tip of the breastbone.

FYI

Compressions are important in CPR, and doing them correctly is tiring. The more tired you are, the less effective your compressions are. If someone else knows CPR, take turns. Switch about every 2 minutes, moving quickly so that the pause in compressions is as short as possible. Remind each other to push down about **1½ inches**, to push at a rate of **at least 100 compressions a minute**, and to let the **chest come back up** to its normal position after each compression.

Definitions and Key Facts

Infants often have healthy hearts. Usually, an infant's heart stops because she can't breathe or is having trouble breathing. As a result, it's very important to give breaths as well as compressions to an infant.

Your breaths need to make the infant's chest rise. When the chest rises, you know the infant has gotten enough air. Compressions are the most important part of CPR. If you are also able to give breaths, you will help the infant even more.

Action: Open the Airway

Before giving breaths, open the airway. Follow these steps to open the airway:

Step	Action
1	Put one hand on the forehead and the fingers of your other hand on the bony part of the infant's chin.
2	Tilt the head back and lift the chin.

Important

When tilting an infant's head, do not push it back too far, because this may block the infant's airway. Avoid pressing the soft part of the neck or under the chin.

Action: Give Breaths

Follow these steps to give breaths to an infant:

Step	Action
1	While holding the infant's airway open, take a normal breath.
2	Cover the infant's mouth and nose with your mouth.
3	**Give 2 breaths** (blow for 1 second each). Watch for **the chest to begin to rise** as you give each breath.

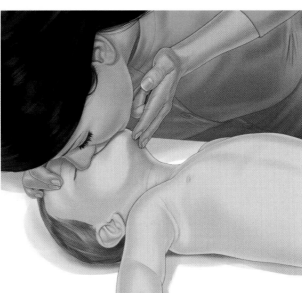

Figure 41. Cover the infant's mouth and nose with your mouth.

If your mouth is too small to cover the infant's mouth and nose, put your mouth over the infant's nose and give breaths through the infant's nose. (You may need to hold the infant's mouth closed to stop air from coming out through the mouth.)

Important

If you give an infant a breath and the chest doesn't rise, reopen the airway by allowing the head to go back to the normal position. Then open the airway again by tilting the head and lifting the chin. Then give another breath. Make sure the chest rises.

Don't interrupt compressions for more than 10 seconds to give breaths. If the chest doesn't rise within 10 seconds, begin pushing hard and pushing fast on the chest again.

Using a Mask

Definitions and Key Facts

Giving breaths to another person is usually quite safe. During CPR there is very little chance that you will catch a disease. Even so, some child care centers require rescuers to have masks.

Masks are made of firm plastic and fit over the infant's mouth or mouth and nose. You may need to put the mask together before you use it.

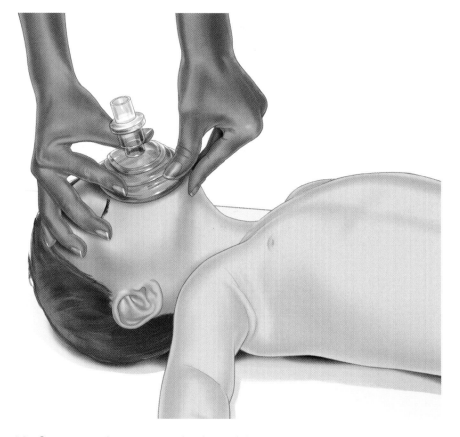

Figure 42. Some people use a mask when giving breaths.

Actions

Follow these steps to give breaths with a mask:

Step	Action
1	Put the mask over the infant's mouth and nose.
2	Tilt the head and lift the chin while pressing the mask against the infant's face. It is important to make an airtight seal between the infant's face and the mask while you lift the chin to keep the airway open.
3	Give 2 breaths. Watch for the chest to begin to rise as you give each breath.

FYI

If the mask has a pointed end

- Put the narrow end of the mask at the top (bridge) of the nose
- The wide end should cover the mouth

Assess and Phone 911

Definitions and Key Facts

Now that you've learned how to give CPR, it's time to learn when to give CPR. If an infant doesn't respond and if that infant isn't breathing or is only gasping, you need to give CPR.

If you are not sure whether to give CPR, go ahead and give it. It's better to give CPR to someone who doesn't need it than not to give it to someone who does need it.

Action: Make Sure the Scene Is Safe

Before you give CPR, make sure the scene is safe. Look for anything nearby that might hurt you. You don't want to hurt yourself.

Action: Tap and Shout

Check if the infant responds. Tap his foot and shout his name. If he doesn't move, make a sound, blink, or otherwise react, he is not responding.

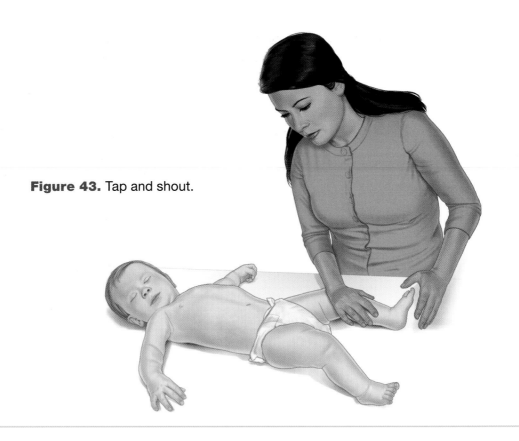

Figure 43. Tap and shout.

Action: Yell for Help Yell for help. If someone comes, have that person phone 911. Whether someone comes or not, check the infant's breathing next.

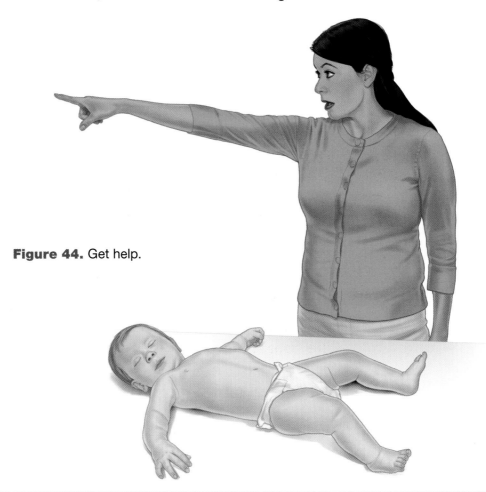

Figure 44. Get help.

Action: Check Breathing

If the infant doesn't respond, check his breathing. If the infant isn't breathing at all or if he is only "gasping," then he needs CPR.

A person who gasps usually appears to be drawing air in very quickly. He may open his mouth and move his jaw, head, or neck. Gasps may appear forceful or weak, and some time may pass between gasps, as they usually happen at a slow rate. The gasp may sound like a snort, snore, or groan. Gasping is not regular or normal breathing. It is a sign of cardiac arrest in someone who doesn't respond.

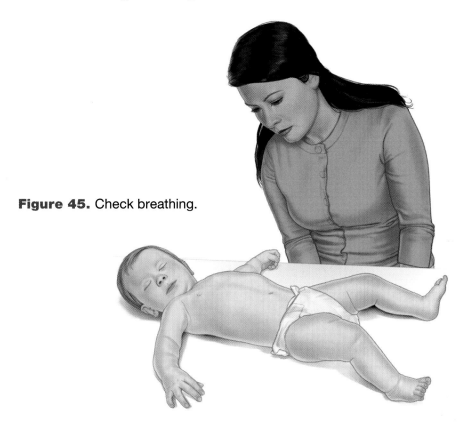

Figure 45. Check breathing.

Put It All Together (*Skill You Will Demonstrate)

Definitions and Key Facts

Since infants' hearts are often healthy and since breathing trouble is often the cause of the infant's heart problem, it's important to get air to the infant as quickly as possible. For this reason, you should give 5 sets of CPR before phoning for help. (If someone else is nearby, send that person to phone for help as soon as possible.)

Compressions are very important and are the core of CPR. Try not to interrupt compressions for more than a few seconds, even when you give breaths.

Action: Give 5 Sets of CPR

When doing CPR on an infant, **give sets of 30 compressions and 2 breaths**. Push down about **1½ inches** at a rate of **at least 100 times a minute**. After each push, let the **chest come back up** to its normal position.

If the infant is not injured and you are alone, after 5 sets of 30 compressions and 2 breaths, you may carry the infant with you to phone 911.

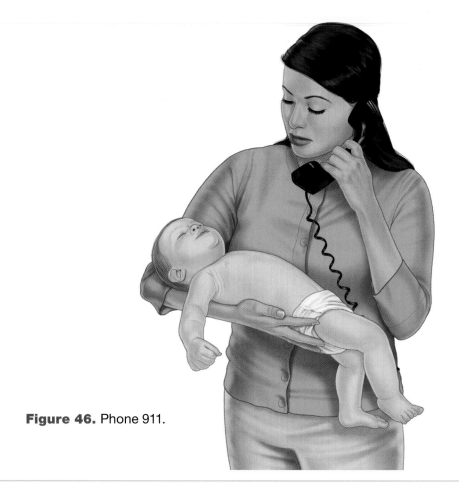

Figure 46. Phone 911.

Action: Phone 911

After 5 sets of CPR, phone 911 if no one has done this yet. Take the infant with you to the phone if possible.

Action: Keep Going

After phoning, keep giving sets of 30 compressions and 2 breaths until the infant begins to respond or until someone with more advanced training arrives and takes over.

FYI: Answering Dispatcher Questions	You need to stay on the phone until the 911 dispatcher (operator) tells you to hang up.

FYI: Answering Dispatcher Questions

You need to stay on the phone until the 911 dispatcher (operator) tells you to hang up.

The dispatcher will ask you about the emergency. She may also tell you how to help the infant until someone with more advanced training arrives and takes over.

Answering the dispatcher's questions will not delay the arrival of help. If you can, take the phone with you or carry the infant with you so that you're with the infant while you talk to the dispatcher.

Action: Infant CPR

No response + No breathing or only gasping = GIVE CPR

Follow these steps for infant CPR:

Step	Action
1	Make sure the scene is safe.
2	Tap and shout.
3	Yell for help.
4	Check breathing.
5	If the infant isn't responding and either isn't breathing or is only gasping, **give 5 sets of 30 compressions and 2 breaths, and then phone 911.**
6	Keep giving **sets of compressions and breaths** until the infant starts to breathe or move, or until someone with more advanced training arrives and takes over.

Important

If another person is with you when you give CPR—or if you can yell for help and get someone to come help you—then send the other person to phone 911 while you start pushing hard and fast and giving breaths. **You give compressions and breaths; the other person phones 911.**

Infant CPR Skills Summary

Step	Action
1	**Make sure the scene is safe.**
2	**Tap and shout.** ▪ Check to see if the infant responds. ▪ If the infant doesn't respond, go to Step 3.
3	**Yell for help.** ▪ See if someone can help you. ▪ Have that person phone 911.
4	**Check breathing.** ▪ Make sure the infant is on a firm, flat surface. If possible, use a surface above the ground. ▪ See if the infant isn't breathing or is only gasping. **No response + No breathing or only gasping = GIVE CPR**
5	**Give CPR. Give 5 sets of 30 compressions and 2 breaths, and then phone 911 (if no one has phoned yet).** ▪ Compressions: 　– Move clothes out of the way. 　– Place 2 fingers just below the nipple line. 　– Push straight down about 1½ inches at a rate of at least 100 compressions a minute. 　– After each compression, let the chest come back up to its normal position. ▪ Breaths: 　– After 30 compressions, open the airway with a head tilt–chin lift. 　– After the airway is open, take a normal breath. 　– Cover the infant's mouth and nose with your mouth. 　– Give 2 breaths (blow for 1 second each). Watch for the chest to begin to rise as you give each breath.
6	**Keep going.** ▪ Keep giving sets of 30 compressions and 2 breaths until the infant starts to breathe or move, or until someone with more advanced training arrives and takes over.

How to Help a Choking Infant

What You Will Learn In this section you'll learn the signs of choking in an infant and how to help a choking infant.

Definitions and Key Facts Choking is when food or another object gets stuck in the airway or throat. The object stops air from getting to the lungs.

Some choking is mild and some is severe. If it's severe, act fast. Get the object out so the infant can breathe.

Topics Covered
- Mild vs Severe Choking
- How to Help a Choking Infant
- How to Help a Choking Infant Who Stops Responding

Mild vs Severe Choking

Action Use the following table to figure out if an infant has mild or severe choking and what you should do.

If the infant	The block in the airway is	And you should
• Can make sounds • Can cough loudly	Mild	• Stand by and let her cough • If you are worried about the infant's breathing, phone 911
• Cannot breathe or • Has a cough that has no sound or • Cannot make a sound	Severe	• Act quickly • Follow the steps to help a choking infant

How to Help a Choking Infant

Definitions and Key Facts

When an infant has severe choking, use back slaps and chest thrusts to help remove the object blocking the airway.

Action: Help a Choking Infant

Follow these steps to help a choking infant:

Step	Action
1	Hold the infant facedown on your forearm. Support the infant's head and jaw with your hand.
2	Give up to **5 back slaps** with the heel of your other hand between the infant's shoulder blades.
3	If the object does not come out after 5 back slaps, turn the infant onto her back, supporting the head.
4	Give up to **5 chest thrusts** using 2 fingers of your other hand to push on the chest in the same place you push during CPR.
5	**Repeat** giving 5 back slaps and 5 chest thrusts until the infant can breathe, cough, or cry or until she stops responding.

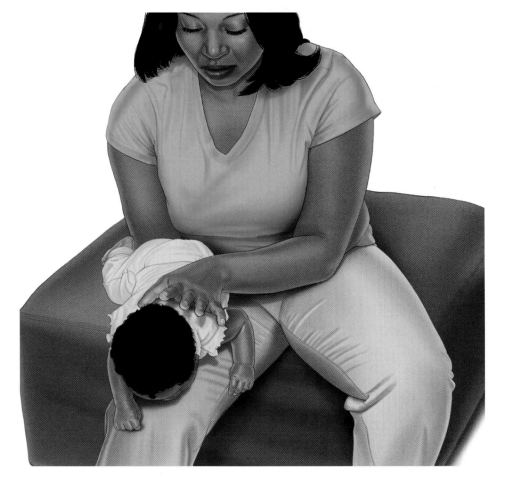

Figure 47. Give up to 5 back slaps.

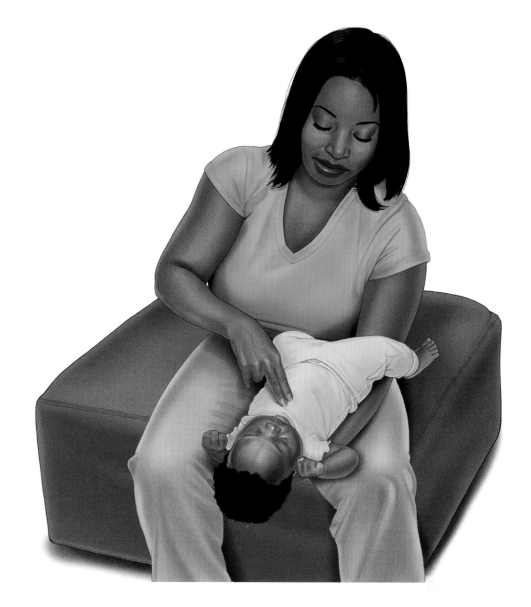

Figure 48. Give up to 5 chest thrusts.

FYI

An infant who has been given back slaps and chest thrusts should be seen by a healthcare provider.

How to Help a Choking Infant Who Stops Responding

Definitions and Key Facts

If you give an infant back slaps and chest thrusts and can't remove the object blocking the airway, the infant will stop responding. Pushing on his chest may force the object out.

Action: Help a Choking Infant Who Stops Responding

Follow these steps if the infant stops responding:

Step	Action
1	Place the infant faceup on a firm, flat surface above the ground, such as a table.
2	Tap and shout.
3	**Yell for help.**
4	**Check breathing.**
5	**Compress the chest 30 times.**
6	After 30 compressions, open the airway. **If you see an object in the mouth, take it out.**
7	**Give 2 breaths.**
8	**Repeat** giving **sets of 30 compressions and 2 breaths**, checking the mouth for objects after each set of compressions.
9	**After 5 sets of 30 compressions and 2 breaths, phone 911.**
10	**Give sets of 30 compressions and 2 breaths**, checking the mouth for objects after each set of compressions until the infant starts to respond or until someone with more advanced training arrives and takes over.

Important

Give only back slaps and chest thrusts to an infant. Giving thrusts to his abdomen could cause serious harm.

If another person is with you when the infant stops responding—or if you can yell for help and get someone to come help you—send the other person to phone 911 while you start pushing hard and fast and giving breaths. **You give compressions and breaths; the other person phones 911.**

CPR and AED for Adults

What You Will Learn	In this section you'll learn when CPR is needed, how to give CPR to an adult, and how to use an AED.
Definitions and Key Facts	For the purpose of this course, an adult is anyone who has gone through or is going through puberty. When in doubt, treat someone as an adult. Someone who "responds" moves, speaks, blinks, or otherwise reacts to you when you tap him and ask if he's OK. Someone who doesn't "respond" does nothing when you tap him and ask if he's OK.
Topics Covered	▪ Give CPR: Compressions and Breaths ▪ Use an AED ▪ Assess and Phone 911 ▪ Put It All Together

Give CPR: Compressions and Breaths

Definitions and Key Facts	CPR has 2 main parts: compressions and giving breaths. Pushing hard and fast on the chest is the most important part of CPR. When you push on the chest, you pump blood to the brain and heart.

Compressions

Definitions and Key Facts	A compression is the act of pushing on the chest. People often don't push hard enough because they're afraid of hurting the victim. An injury is unlikely, but it is better than death. It's better to push too hard than not hard enough.

Action: Push Hard and Push Fast

Follow these steps to push hard and push fast:

Step	Actions
1	Make sure the person is lying on his back on a firm, flat surface.
2	Move clothes out of the way.
3	Put the heel of one hand on the lower half of the breastbone. Put the heel of your other hand on top of the first hand.
4	Push straight down **at least 2 inches** at a rate of **at least 100 compressions a minute.**
5	After each compression, let the **chest come back up** to its normal position.

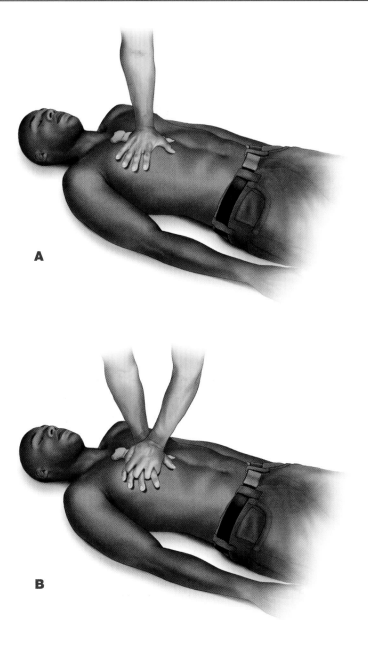

Figure 49. Compressions. **A,** Put the heel of one hand on the lower half of the breastbone. **B,** Put the other hand on top of the first hand.

FYI

Compressions are very important, and doing them correctly is tiring. The more tired you are, the less effective your compressions are. If someone else knows CPR, take turns. Switch about every 2 minutes, moving quickly to keep the pause between compressions as short as possible. Remind each other to push down **at least 2 inches,** push at a rate of **at least 100 compressions a minute,** and let **the chest come back up** to its normal position after each compression.

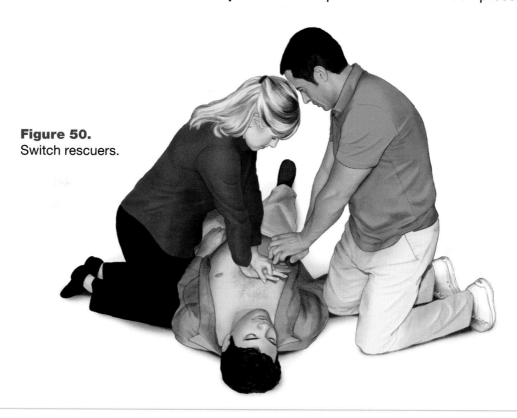

Figure 50.
Switch rescuers.

Give Breaths

Definitions and Key Facts

Compressions are the most important part of CPR. If you're also able to give breaths, you will help even more. Your breaths need to make the chest rise. When the chest rises, you know the person has taken in enough air.

Action: Open the Airway

Before giving breaths, open the airway. Follow these steps to open the airway:

Step	Action
1	Put one hand on the forehead and the fingers of your other hand on the bony part of the chin.
2	Tilt the head back and lift the chin.

Important	Avoid pressing on the soft part of the neck or under the chin.

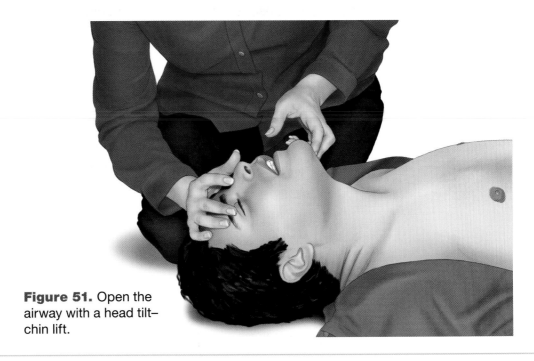

Figure 51. Open the airway with a head tilt–chin lift.

Action: Give Breaths

Follow these steps to give breaths to an adult:

Step	Action
1	While holding the airway open, pinch the nose closed.
2	Take a breath. Cover the person's mouth with your mouth.
3	Give 2 breaths (blow for 1 second each). **Watch for the chest to begin to rise** as you give each breath.

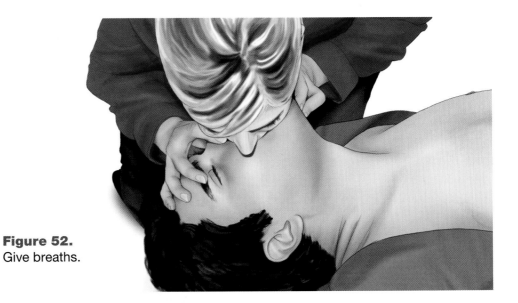

Figure 52. Give breaths.

Important

If you give someone a breath and the chest doesn't rise, allow the head to go back to its normal position. Then open the airway again by tilting the head and lifting the chin. Then give another breath. Make sure the chest rises.

Don't interrupt compressions for more than 10 seconds to give breaths. If the chest doesn't rise within 10 seconds, begin pushing hard and pushing fast on the chest again.

Definitions and Key Facts

Giving breaths to another person is usually quite safe. During CPR there is very little chance that you will catch a disease. Even so, some child care centers require rescuers to have masks.

Masks are made of firm plastic and fit over the ill or injured person's mouth or mouth and nose. You may need to put the mask together before you use it.

Figure 53. Some people use a mask when giving breaths.

Actions

Follow these steps to give breaths with a mask:

Step	Action
1	Put the mask over the person's mouth and nose.
2	Tilt the head and lift the chin while pressing the mask against the person's face. It is important to make an airtight seal between the person's face and the mask while you lift the chin to keep the airway open.
3	Give 2 breaths (blow for 1 second each). Watch for the chest to begin to rise as you give each breath.

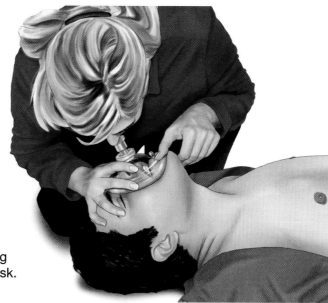

Figure 54. Giving breaths with a mask.

If the mask has a pointed end

- Put the narrow end of the mask at the top (bridge) of the nose
- Position the wide end so it covers the mouth

Use an AED

Definitions and Key Facts

Sometimes a heart doesn't work right. An AED is a machine with a computer in it that can shock the heart and help it work properly again. If you start CPR right away and then use an AED within a few minutes, you will have the best chance of saving a life.

AEDs are safe, accurate, and easy to use. The AED will figure out if the person needs a shock and will tell you to give one if needed. It will even tell you when to make sure that no one is touching the person. The pads used to shock the person have a diagram showing you where to place them. Follow the diagram.

The most common ways to turn on an AED are to push an "ON" button or lift the lid of the AED. Once you turn on the AED, it will tell you everything you need to do.

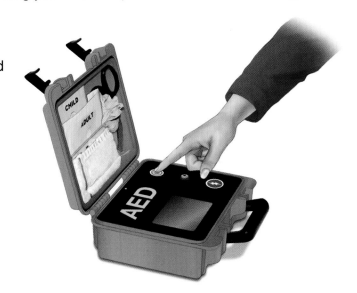

Figure 55. An AED.

Actions

Use an AED if someone doesn't respond and isn't breathing or is only gasping. Follow these steps for using an AED:

Step	Action
1	Turn the AED on.
2	Follow the prompts you see and hear.

Important

If you have access to an AED, use it as quickly as possible. Make sure no one is touching the victim just before you push the "SHOCK" button. If you can't find an AED quickly, then start CPR. Push hard and push fast.

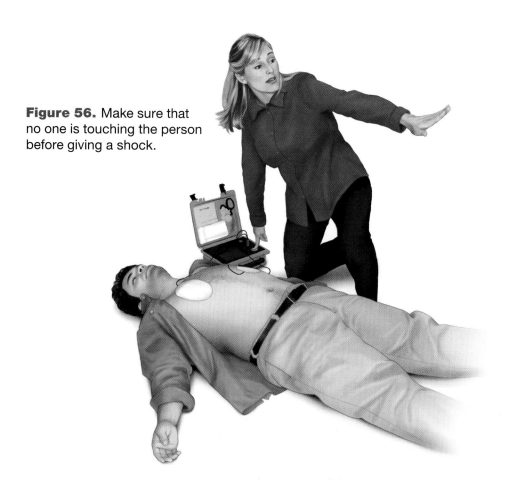

Figure 56. Make sure that no one is touching the person before giving a shock.

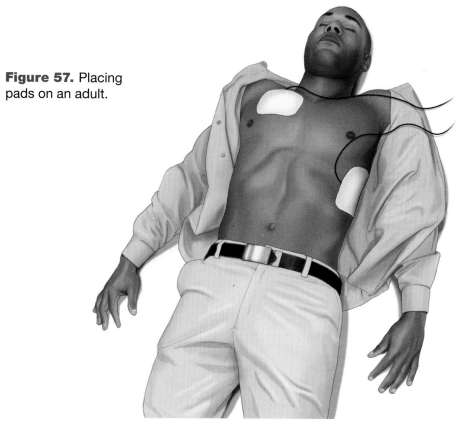

Figure 57. Placing pads on an adult.

Definitions and Key Facts

If a person doesn't respond and if that person isn't breathing or is only gasping, then you need to give CPR.

If you are not sure whether to give CPR, go ahead and give it. It's better to give CPR to someone who doesn't need it than not to give it to someone who does need it.

Action: Make Sure the Scene Is Safe

Before you assess the need for CPR, make sure the scene is safe. Look for anything nearby that might hurt you. You don't want to hurt yourself.

Action: Tap and Shout

Check if the person responds. Tap him and shout, "Are you OK?" If he doesn't move, speak, blink, or otherwise react, then he is not responding.

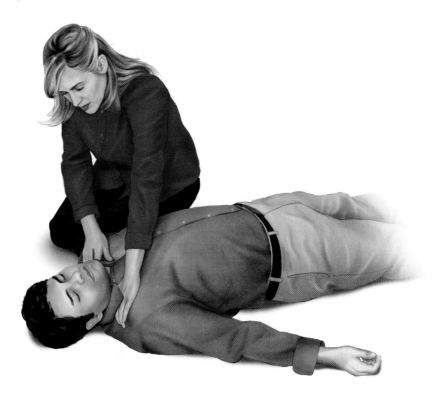

Figure 58. Tap and shout.

Action: Phone 911 and Get AED

If the person doesn't respond, it's important to get help. You or someone else (yell for help if you need to) should phone 911. Get an AED, if available.

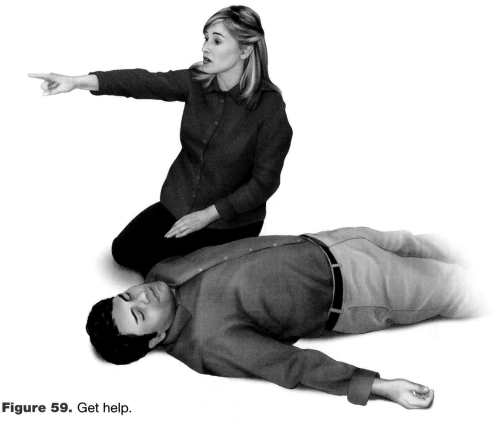

Figure 59. Get help.

Important

Stay on the phone until the 911 dispatcher (operator) tells you to hang up. Answering the dispatcher's questions will not delay the arrival of help.

Action: Check Breathing

If the person doesn't respond, check his breathing. If the person isn't breathing at all or if he is only "gasping," then he needs CPR.

A person who gasps usually appears to be drawing air in very quickly. He may open his mouth and move the jaw, head, or neck. Gasps may appear forceful or weak, and some time may pass between gasps because they usually happen at a slow rate. The gasp may sound like a snort, snore, or groan. Gasping is not regular or normal breathing. It is a sign of cardiac arrest in someone who doesn't respond.

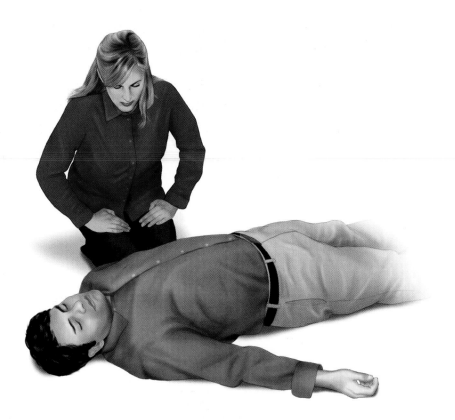

Figure 60. Check breathing.

FYI

If the person is breathing but is not responding, roll him onto his side and wait for someone with more advanced training to arrive and take over. Placing someone in the side position helps keep the airway clear in the event the person vomits. If the person stops breathing or is only gasping, you will need to roll him onto his back and assess the need for CPR.

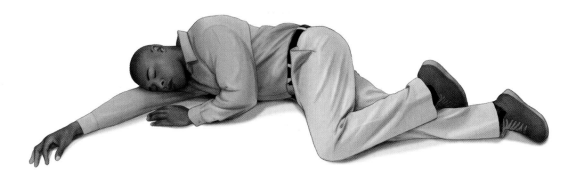

Figure 61. Side position.

Definitions and Key Facts

When doing CPR, you **give sets of 30 compressions and 2 breaths**. Push straight down **at least 2 inches** at a rate of **at least 100 times a minute**. After each compression, let the **chest come back up** to its normal position.

Try not to interrupt compressions for more than 10 seconds, even when you give breaths.

Action: Adult CPR

Follow these steps for adult CPR:

Step	Action
1	Make sure the scene is safe.
2	Tap and shout.
3	Yell for help. You or someone else should phone 911 and get the AED.
4	Check breathing.
5	If the person isn't breathing or is only gasping, give CPR.
6	Give **30 compressions** at a **rate of at least 100 a minute** and a depth of **at least 2 inches**. After each compression, **let the chest come back up** to its normal position.
7	Open the airway and give **2 breaths**.
8	Keep giving sets of 30 compressions and 2 breaths until the AED arrives, the person starts to respond, or trained help arrives and takes over.

The following table summarizes differences between adult and child CPR:

What's Different	What to Do for an Adult	What to Do for a Child
When to phone 911	Phone after checking for a response.	Phone after giving 5 sets of compressions and breaths if you are alone.
Using an AED	Use the adult pads.	• Look for a child key or switch. • Use the child pads. • If there are no child pads, use the adult pads. • If you use adult pads, make sure the pads don't touch each other.
Compression depth	Push down at least 2 inches.	Push down about 2 inches.

Adult CPR AED Skills Summary

Step	Action
1	**Make sure the scene is safe.**
2	**Tap and shout.** ▪ Check to see if the person responds. ▪ If the person doesn't respond, go to Step 3.
3	**Get help.** ▪ Yell for help. ▪ Have the person who comes phone 911 and get an AED. ▪ If no one can help, phone 911 and get an AED. Use it.
4	**Check breathing.** ▪ Make sure the person is on a firm, flat surface. ▪ Check breathing. ▪ If the person isn't breathing at all or is only gasping, give CPR. **No response** + **No breathing or only gasping** = **GIVE CPR**
5	**Push and give breaths. Give 30 compressions and 2 breaths.** ▪ Compressions: – Move clothes out of the way. – Put the heel of one hand on the lower half of the breastbone. Put the heel of your other hand on top of the first hand. – Push straight down at least 2 inches at a rate of at least 100 compressions a minute. – After each compression, let the chest come back up to its normal position. – Compress the chest 30 times. ▪ Breaths: – After 30 compressions, open the airway with a head tilt–chin lift. – After the airway is open, take a normal breath. – Pinch the nose shut. Cover the mouth with your mouth. – Give 2 breaths (blow for 1 second each). Watch for the chest to begin to rise as you give each breath. ▪ AED: – Use it as soon as you have it. – Turn it on by lifting the lid or pressing the "ON" button. – Follow the prompts.
6	**Keep going.** ▪ Keep giving sets of compressions and breaths until the person starts to breathe or move, or until someone with more advanced training arrives and takes over.

How to Help a Choking Adult

What You Will Learn

In this section we'll cover

- Mild vs Severe Choking
- How to Help a Choking Adult
- How to Help a Choking Adult Who Stops Responding

Definitions and Key Facts

Choking is when food or another object gets stuck in the airway in the throat. The object stops air from getting to the lungs.

Some choking is mild and some is severe. If it's severe, act fast. Get the object out so the person can breathe.

Topics Covered

- Mild vs Severe Choking
- How to Help a Choking Adult
- How to Help a Choking Adult Who Stops Responding

Mild vs Severe Choking

Action

Use the following table to figure out if someone has mild or severe choking and what you should do:

If someone	The block in the airway is	And you should
• Can make sounds • Can cough loudly	Mild	• Stand by and let her cough • If worried about her breathing, phone 911
• Cannot breathe or • Has a cough that has no sound or • Cannot talk or make a sound or • Makes the choking sign	Severe	• Act quickly • Follow the steps to help a choking adult

FYI: The Choking Sign	If someone is choking, he might use the choking sign (holding the neck with one or both hands).

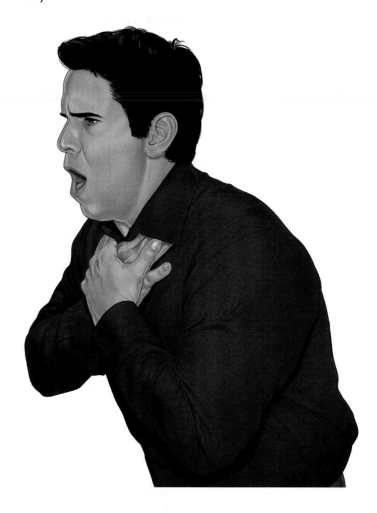

Figure 62. The choking sign: holding the neck with one or both hands.

How to Help a Choking Adult

Definitions and Key Facts	When someone has severe choking, give thrusts slightly above the belly button. These thrusts are sometimes called the Heimlich maneuver. Like a cough, each thrust pushes air from the lungs. This can help remove an object that is blocking the airway.

Action: Help a Choking Adult	Follow these steps to help a choking adult:

Step	Action
1	If you think someone is choking, ask, "Are you choking?" If he nods yes, tell him you are going to help.
2	**Get behind him.** Wrap your arms around him so that your hands are in front.

(continued)

(continued)

Step	Action
3	**Make a fist** with one hand.
4	Put the thumb side of your fist slightly above his belly button and well below the breastbone.
5	**Grasp the fist with your other hand** and give quick upward thrusts into his abdomen.
6	**Give thrusts** until the object is forced out and he can breathe, cough, or talk, or until he stops responding.

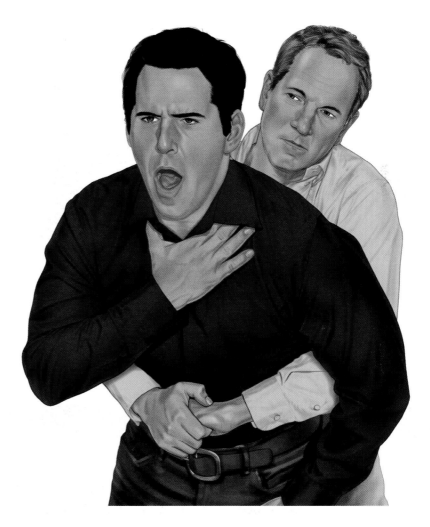

Figure 63. Helping someone who is choking.

Action: Help a Choking Large Person or Pregnant Woman

If someone is choking and is in the late stages of pregnancy or is very large and you can't wrap your arms fully around the waist, give thrusts on the chest instead of thrusts on the abdomen.

Follow the same steps except for the location where you place your arms and hands. Put your arms under the armpits and your hands on the lower half of the breastbone. Pull straight back to give the chest thrusts.

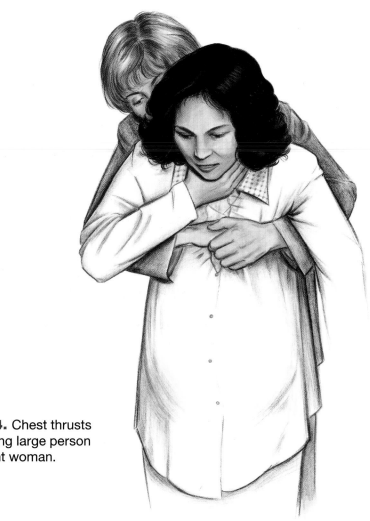

Figure 64. Chest thrusts on a choking large person or pregnant woman.

FYI

Any person who has received thrusts should tell her healthcare provider.

How to Help a Choking Adult Who Stops Responding

Definitions and Key Facts

If you give someone thrusts but can't remove the object blocking the airway, the person will stop responding.

Action

Follow these steps if the adult stops responding:

Step	Action
1	Check if he needs CPR. Give it if needed.
2	After each set of 30 compressions, open the airway. If you see an object in the mouth, take it out.
3	Continue CPR until he speaks, moves, or breathes or until someone with more advanced training arrives and takes over.

Conclusion

Congratulations on completing this course.

Practice your skills often. This will keep them fresh and help you prepare for an emergency. It's important to phone the emergency number (or 911) when an emergency arises. The operator also may be able to remind you what to do.

Contact the American Heart Association if you want more information on first aid, CPR, or AED training. You can visit **www.heart.org/cpr** or call 1-877-AHA-4CPR (877-242-4277) to find a class near you.

Even if you don't remember all the steps exactly, it is important for you to try. Any help, even if it isn't perfect, is better than no help at all.

Reference Materials

Sample First Aid Action Plan

This is a sample only. The actions listed are not for use for an actual child. Always follow instructions from the child's caregiver or physician.

Seizure First Aid Action Plan for
Jimmy Childs

Date of Birth: June 3, 2009
Parents: John and Mary Childs
Parents' Contact Phone Number: 999-452-5555 or 999-321-4444
Jimmy's Physician (for seizures): Dr. A. J. Nest, 999-322-3333

Medical Condition: Seizures

Jimmy Childs has a condition known as epilepsy. He may have a seizure that will cause him to no longer respond and to have uncontrolled movements of his arms and legs. These seizures usually last a short time. These seizures may last for a longer time or occur with one followed quickly by another.

Possible triggers:

Bright, flashing lights may trigger a seizure.

Staff members trained to give medications:

1. Jean Oro
2. Martha Garcia

Staff members trained in First Aid and CPR AED:

1. Jean Oro
2. Martha Garcia
3. Jan Door
4. Stephen Glass

Actions

Follow First Aid actions for seizures as you have been trained to do.

If a seizure lasts longer than 4 minutes or if Jimmy has one seizure followed soon after by another, follow these actions. Only give medicines if you are one of the staff members trained to do so:

1. Have one staff member phone 911. Let them know a trained staff member will be administering rectal medicine prescribed by Jimmy's physician.
2. The trained staff member will obtain Jimmy Childs' medicine from the office cabinet. Have another staff member quickly check the label to ensure it is Jimmy's medicine.
3. If Jimmy is still having a seizure, give one dose of diazepam rectal gel using the steps printed on the package.
4. As soon as possible, phone John or Mary Childs.
5. A first aid–trained staff member will stay with Jimmy at all times.
6. If John or Mary Childs does not arrive by the time the ambulance is ready to transport Jimmy, instruct the emergency medical personnel to take Jimmy to Oceanview Children's Hospital.
7. After Jimmy is in the care of emergency medical personnel, write a summary of what happened before the seizure, during the seizure, after the medication was given, and after the seizure stopped. Provide a copy of this to John or Mary Childs.

Sample First Aid Kit

The following table lists sample first aid kit contents. This is a kit that follows ANSI standards. Different child care centers may have different requirements.

Item	Minimum Size or Volume	Quantity per Package	Unit Package Size
List of important local emergency telephone numbers, including police, fire department, EMS, and poison control center*			
Absorbent compress	32 sq. in.	1	1
Adhesive bandage	1 in. × 3 in.	16	1
Adhesive tape	2.5 yd. (total)	1 or 2	1 or 2
Antibiotic treatment	0.14 fl. oz.	6	1
Antiseptic swab	0.14 fl. oz.	10	1
Antiseptic wipe	1 in. × 1 in.	10	1
Antiseptic towelette	24 sq. in.	10	1
Bandage compress (2 in.)	2 in. × 36 in.	4	1
Bandage compress (3 in.)	3 in. × 60 in.	2	1
Bandage compress (4 in.)	4 in. × 72 in.	1	1
Burn dressing	4 in. × 4 in.	1	1 or 2
Burn treatment	1/32 oz.	6	1
CPR barrier		1	1 or 2
Cold pack	4 in. × 5 in.	1	2
Eye covering, with means of attachment	2.9 sq. in.	2	1
Eye/skin wash	4 fl. oz. total	1	2
Gloves		2 pairs	1 or 2
Roller bandage (4 in.)	4 in. × 4 yd.	1	1
Roller bandage (2 in.)	2 in. × 4 yd.	2	1
Sterile pad	3 in. × 3 in.	4	1
Triangular bandage	40 in. × 40 in. × 56 in.	1	1
Heartsaver Pediatric First Aid Quick Reference Guide*			

Items meet the ANSI Z308.1-2009 standard, except those marked with an asterisk.

Summary of CPR and AED for Adults, Children, and Infants

Action	Adult and Older Child (has gone through or is going through puberty)	Child (1 to puberty)	Infant (less than 1 year old)
Check for response	Tap and shout		
Phone your emergency response number (or 911)	Phone your emergency response number (or 911) as soon as you find that the person does not respond	Phone your emergency response number (or 911) after giving 5 sets of 30 compressions and 2 breaths (if you are alone)	
• **Give compressions**			
• **Compression location**	Lower half of the breastbone		Just below the nipple line
• **Compression method**	2 hands	1 or 2 hands	2 fingers
• **Compression depth**	At least 2 inches	About 2 inches	About 1½ inches
• **Compression rate**	At least 100 a minute		
• **Sets of compressions and breaths**	30:2		
Open the airway Use a head tilt–chin lift	Head tilt–chin lift		Head tilt–chin lift (do not tilt the head back too far)
Check breathing	Look for only gasping or no breathing (take at least 5 seconds but no more than 10 seconds)		
Start CPR	Give sets of 30 compressions and 2 breaths (1 second each)		
AED • **Press the "ON" button or open the lid**	Use the AED as soon as it arrives		
• **Attach pads to the person's bare chest**	Use adult pads	Use child pads/key/switch if child is between 1 and 8 years old or adult pads if child is 8 or older	
• **Follow the AED prompts**			

Index

READING, WRITING and CPR

High school is full of life lessons. It should also include lifesaving lessons.

It's time for students to learn CPR before they graduate — a change that would put thousands of qualified lifesavers on our streets every year.

CPR given right away could save you, your relatives or your neighbors if you should become one of the 360,000 people who have an out-of-hospital cardiac arrest each year.

Help support state laws that will ensure all students are trained in lifesaving CPR before they graduate from high school.

Pledge your support at becprsmart.org.

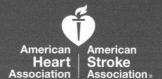

American Heart Association | American Stroke Association

you're the cure

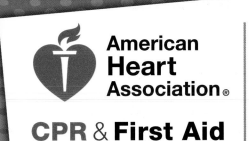 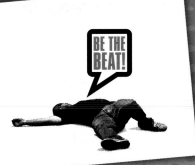

Be the Beat!

We're Training a Team of Heart Heroes

Be the Beat is a free online cardiac arrest awareness website that offers games, music videos and giveaways that teach the simple steps to save a life – while having fun!

Cardiac arrest can strike anyone, anywhere – and victims' chances of survival depend on the people around them. If you see a teen or adult suddenly collapse, calling 911, starting CPR and using an AED can double – or even triple – a victim's chance of survival.

Don't Just Stand There!

Visit **www.bethebeat.heart.org**. It only takes a few minutes to learn about these lifesaving steps and join the movement of teen lifesavers who are ready to step in and Be the Beat if they ever need to.

bethebeat.heart.org

American Heart Association Heartsaver® courses are for individuals with limited or no medical training who need a course completion card for job, regulatory or other requirements.

eLEARNING COURSES

eLearning courses offer the flexibility to complete the online portion (Part 1) at the student's own pace at home or work.

Course Name	Content Taught	Estimated Time	Course Completion Card or Certificate
Heartsaver® First Aid Online Part 1	Basic first aid skills	1-1.5 hours online; up to 1 hour for skills session	Course Completion Card; valid for 2 years
Heartsaver® First Aid CPR AED Online Part 1	Basic first aid skills and adult CPR and AED use (optional infant and child modules)	1.5-2.5 hours online; up to 1 hour for skills session	Course Completion Card; valid for 2 years
Heartsaver® CPR AED Online Part 1	Adult CPR and AED use (optional infant and child modules)	30 minutes–1 hour online; up to 1 hour for skills session	Course Completion Card; valid for 2 years
Heartsaver® Bloodborne Pathogens Online	How to protect yourself and others from exposure to blood or blood-containing materials	1 hour online; skills session not required; must be paired with site-specific training	Participation Certificate; valid for 1 year

CLASSROOM COURSES

Classroom-based courses are ideal for those who prefer group interaction and feedback during class from an AHA Instructor.

Course Name	Content Taught	Estimated Time	Course Completion Card or Certificate
Heartsaver® First Aid	Basic first aid skills	2–3 hours	Course Completion Card; valid for 2 years
Heartsaver® First Aid CPR AED	Basic first aid skills and adult CPR and AED use (optional infant and child modules)	5–7 hours	Course Completion Card; valid for 2 years
Heartsaver® CPR AED	Adult CPR and AED use (optional infant and child modules)	3–4 hours	Course Completion Card; valid for 2 years
Heartsaver® Bloodborne Pathogens*	How to protect yourself and others from exposure to blood or blood-containing materials	1 hour; must be paired with site-specific training	Participation Certificate; valid for 1 year

Available in Spanish.